Robfto Alugon
4/13/96

FOODS THAT HEAL

REVERSE AGING AND
EXTEND YOUR LIFESPAN

AMERICAN PUBLISHING CORP.

IMPORTANT NOTICE

This manual is intended as a reference volume only, not as a medical guide or a reference for self treatment. You should always seek com-petent medical advice from a doctor if you suspect a problem.

This book is intended as educational device to keep you informed of the latest medical knowledge. It is not intended to serve as a substi-tute for changing the treatment advice of your doctor. You should never make medical changes without first consulting your doctor.

Additional copies of this book may be purchased directly from the publisher. To order, please enclose $16.95 plus $3 postage and han-dling. Send to:

FOODS THAT HEAL
American Publishing Corporation
Book Distribution Center
Post Box 15196
Montclair, CA 19763

Printed in the United States of America

0 9 8 7 6 5 4 3 2

ISBN NO. 0-9638596-3-3

Foods That Heal
Reverse Aging and Extend Your Lifespan!

Table of Contents

INTRODUCTION

Through proper nutrition I hope to live to be 100. After all, my grandmother made it to 97, and she was following dietary ideas she had gotten long before I was born. With all that we know now about diet and nutrition we should be able to do a little better than our grandparents. People have always talked about the benefits of a good diet and the harm that a bad diet can do. I just think that we can do better today. The problem with most dietary advice has been that a good diet was also a boring diet. If you only knew of one food that was good for, say, high blood pressure, you would get tired of it after a while and go back to eating something you enjoyed no matter what happened to you. I want to get away from that by giving you a variety of foods that can be used for most medical problems.

But that is kind of a personal bias of mine. I always look for a variety of ways to get where I want to be, and since I find the healing hints hidden in diet totally fascinating, why shouldn't I spend some time on finding foods that will do the same job as a medication that I buy through a doctor or pharmacist? Through my own readings on diet I can find out which foods out of the super market can keep me happy and healthy for all the years of my life, as well as add many years to my life along the way? American markets sell thousands of foods, and many of them are the original sources of the medicines that the medical companies sell us. All that we need is some knowledge and we can go right to the source.

If you pay any attention at all to the nutrition information in the newspapers you have already heard that whole grains are good for you, fish is good for you, red meat can be bad for you, you need to limit your fat intake, and a whole bunch of other things that may be true, but which are so disorganized that you really don't know which foods to pick to keep healthy or heal an illness, and which to avoid.

That is the purpose of this book. To give you a road map among all of the foods in the market. For instance, did you know that whole grain breads are one of the clues to living longer, or that you should eat fish to prevent cancer. These are only a couple of the ideas that we will be exploring, along with a lot of helpful hints as to why good nutrition will keep you healthier than poor nutrition.

You see, most people don't consider themselves to have a bad diet. They know that they have a few problems with the things they eat, but that doesn't mean that they have a bad diet. Well, actually it does. If every meal that you have contains foods that injure your health, then you have a bad diet.

That is why I spend part of each topic discussing what foods to avoid, part giving you some guides as to what foods should be included, and part of the time talking about supplements and exercise, or anything else that might be useful to you to make you healthier.

To make it easier to find information about your own personal interests the book has been divided into topic areas. Under aging, for instance, we take a look at whether you can reverse aging with anti-aging foods? How aging and disease are caused largely by the foods we eat. An herb with a 5,000 year history of countering aging problems. Coenzyme Q10, from soybean and corn oils, a miracle anti-aging food? Strengthen the gland that controls aging through diet. The vitamin that combats oxidation at the cell level to counter aging. A tea to help you feel and look younger.

I don't even try to cover every topic in every area, but I do make an effort to give you some information about all of the problems that I have seen recently as major health concerns. I want to get you started on the right road to good health through nutrition, but I need your help in that you are willing to read what I have put together here, and to put it into practice.

ADVERTISING

I have chosen to start this book with a few words on advertising. Magazines and TV advertise over-the-counter medications, doctors, and even hospitals for the treatment of many illnesses. They all promise relief and cure, and none are entirely honest. If they were honest they would give you the likelihood of failure as well as success, and they would tell you how good other products and other approaches other than theirs are. But it is not their business to be honest, it is their business to make money, and that is why you will never hear more than half of a story from any advertisement. I want you to be aware of the lies you may hear, and of why you are told them. This information will help you make better, and better informed, choices of what you should do for your health.

LIES TO WATCH OUT FOR, AND WHY MEDICINE ONLY TRIES TO TREAT YOU

Advertising medical services largely consists of lies. While an ad may tell you to get treatment anywhere, what they really mean is that you should only get treatment from them. The doctor who advertises presents himself as the best possible doctor for the service he is offering whether it is facelifts or treatment for heart disease. Medications are presented the same way, and you are never told that a headache or stomach ache cannot be cured with a simple dose of their product. While these medications may be effective for what they do, they are not the only treatments available, and are often not the best. For instance headaches can be treated just as well with a simple acupressure technique in which one person squeezes the skin between the thumb and fore-finger of another person on both hands tightly, releasing it slowly, to relieve headaches instantly and without medication of any kind. This simple technique is free, and can even be performed by a person on himself You will never see it presented in an ad for headache treatments since no one will make a profit from it.

But this brings up the other point of advertising, it promotes treatment and not prevention. The treatment may be intended to cure, or just to relieve symptoms, but it is not given as an idea by which you can prevent the development of an illness. Now why should medical advertising take this approach, and not the one of prevention? It is because treatment must be paid for, when delivered in the form of medication, and prevention is essentially free. That is it is free of profits to the medical and health industry. If controlling your weight will prevent you from getting arthritis, a seller of arthritis medicine is not going to recommend losing weight along with his pain relief medication.

Prevention, and treatment through such means as exercise and diet, are largely up to the decision of the individual. Prevention has the added advantage in that you don't even know many of the problems you have prevented when you take care of yourself, and manage your diet to your best interests. Again, prevention will not cure a disease that you may have, but it will help you control it. I want this book to place some of the means into your hands of preventing the illnesses you may be concerned about, and of assisting in, or self-treating, many of the diseases you may acquire. To these ends I will include as much information as possible so that you may make the decisions of what and how to treat in the ways that best fits your abilities and your needs.

AGING

Aging is inevitable for those of us who survive. But aging is not the same as getting sick. Certainly we all die, but why should we spend years in sickness and pain while we live just because we are getting older. Prevention gets harder over the years since bad habits and accidents add up on us to create chronic illnesses, but even these can be helped with the proper care. This book is concerned with using the most effective diet in order to care for each of the problems we encounter. We will see how diet can hold off the diseases of aging, and even reverse some of them that do catch up with us. We will also see how diet causes disease over time. Foods have been looked for over many centuries to counter the problems of aging, and new nutrients, such as coenzyme Q10, have been discovered that may be the miracle anti-aging food we all want. Along the way you will even be introduced to a vitamin that combats oxidation, and a tea that can help to rejuvenate you so that you both feel and look younger.

CAN YOU REALLY REVERSE AGING WITH ANTI-AGING FOODS?

You can't reverse age, but you can reverse many of the effects of getting older. What do people fear as they grow older? That they will be sick all of the time, that they will be unable to do the things they like, that they will be in pain, and that they just plain won't feel good. Death is not really something that we should fear as we grow older any more than we fear it when we are younger, and other than making arrangements for our affairs when we can, it is not worth worrying about. This brings up the first order of business in reversing the effects of aging, worry.

Worry itself, whether over age, health, or death, is a worse illness than any of these. Worry can prevent you from doing any of the things that you want to, no matter what your physical abilities. So the first step in reversing the effects of aging is to banish, or minimize worry. To start with, worry never solves any problem, only action solves problems. If you have a problem, act to solve it. If your health is bad, do something to get better or feel better. If the problem is with a friend or family member worry will just prevent you from helping them, or even from supporting them as you are best able.

Now these are psychological solutions to one of the problems of aging, but it would be nice to have some dietary solutions as well. Something you can do everyday, and largely without thinking about it, which will help you overcome your physical problems.

Many of the effects of aging can be reversed through relieving the symptoms, and even occasionally by getting cures. Food can contribute to this process since foods contain the source of many of the drugs that are used to treat these diseases, and a good diet can even help you to feel younger and more energetic.

HOW AGING AND DISEASE ARE CAUSED LARGELY BY THE FOODS WE EAT

Most Americans do not die of infectious diseases such as malaria and the plague. What kills us are the diseases of aging such as heart disease and cancer. These diseases are largely the result of poor diets, and by improving what we eat we can minimize the risk we face in getting them. Have you ever wondered why older people suffer from more of these kind of disease than younger people? It is not just aging, it is that they take a long time to get started, and the longer we live the more likely we are that our bad eating habits are going to catch up to us and give us a disease that may eventually kill us.

A few examples of the diseases of aging and how they are caused by eating habits can begin with high blood pressure. High blood pressure usually results from a combination of a lack of exercise and of having too much fat in the diet. Americans are notorious for having a very high fat intake which starts us down the road to high blood pressure before we are 20 in many cases. Of course for older Americans the problem is how to reverse this problem once it has developed, and the best way to begin is by cutting out as much fat as possible so that the problem doesn't get any worse than it already is.

Another little side effect is diabetes, which tends to become much more common in older persons. Diabetes is known to be associated with obesity, which is caused by high fat and sugar in the diet. Evidence for this is easy to find since mild cases of diabetes are often treated, and even cured through low fat and low sugar diets.

Cancer is a big one, although it is not the problem that heart disease is. The cause of lung cancer has long been named as smoking, and skin cancer is caused largely through exposure to the sun. While some other cancers do not have specified causes, many types of cancer are known to be prevented through the use of broccoli in the diet. Now if you are looking at broccoli for cancer prevention, also keep in mind that broccoli is the same thing as cauliflower. In fields where one is grown the other is often found growing from the same seeds.

These are just a few of the examples of diets where food has caused diseases of aging, and of how diet can be used to cure them. Sometimes it is nothing more than finding out the cause, such as fat, and then just cutting it out. In many other cases you will need to also find a food that can cure the problem along with getting rid of the cause. Who knows, maybe smokers who have put a lot of broccoli into their diets are saving themselves from cancer. Only time will tell, but if I were a smoker I would rather take a chance on eating broccoli than on the hope that the smoking would not hurt me.

AN HERB WITH A 5,000 YEAR HISTORY OF COUNTERING AGING PROBLEMS

One of the oldest methods used by man to counter aging is the Chinese herb ginseng. If you are not familiar with it, it seems like the Chinese believe that ginseng will cure anything. Of course their claims are not that broad, but they do firmly believe that it lengthens life and gives energy to those who use it regularly. There is even medical evidence for these claims since ginseng promotes a healthy immune system, it helps you fight off disease. If you are healthier you will also have fewer aches and pains and live longer as well, so ginseng is beginning to sound like a pretty good form of countering aging problems. Ginseng has also been looked at as a cancer treatment, but to be effective it must be combined with other medicines or herbs.

It is good to know that ginseng seems to have no toxic qualities, and dosage does not have to be carefully watched. For best effect it is recommended that you take ginseng 3 or 4 times over the course of a day. This will keep the levels of active ingredients at a high level in your body. Something else that you want to be aware of though is that there are different kinds of ginseng. Even though it is always thought of as a Chinese medicine, a lot of ginseng is also grown in the United States. Studies have found some difference in the different sources of ginseng, but which is best is up to you. Most of the ginseng sold in this country is from Korea, and some in the form of little bags of pellets that can be dissolved in water or tea. American ginseng is also sold, but at a higher price, and it may even be possible to find Chinese or Taiwanese ginseng, but I have always used the Korean form and been happy with it. The cost varies a lot by the kind of store you get it in. On the west coast 100 packets of ginseng should cost less than $10, although I have seen higher prices. Most of the time I can find it for around $7 a 100 in the Korean form.

Using ginseng brings up one more little problem, what is the best way to take it. If you are not used to it, many people say that it tastes like dirt, and I suppose the very earthy taste of it might seem like that. After all, ginseng is a root, and seems to retain a lot of the taste of the soil it's grown in. If you think that only Americans feel that way about the taste you shouldn't let it bother you. Asians even say the same thing, so that if you don't like it because of the taste don't let it bother you. Ginseng can also be found in capsule form so that you don't have to taste it, but the cost is higher. Personally I prefer to take ginseng in warm water with sugar or sweetener, but I have gotten use to the taste. You might try adding it to tea or coffee if you don't like it straight, or just resorting to the capsules.

In any case ginseng is a 5,000 year old herb that billions of Chinese, and other Asians, have used to counter the effects of aging, and firmly believe in. I tend to think that they have not been fooling themselves all of these years, and that what they believe has a lot of truth to it. Personally I like to have a cup of ginseng tea on a regular basis, and I know that I always feel better when I do. The cost is not great, and the benefits are genuine, if personal experience can be the judge. I recommend it, and I think that everyone should give it a 6 month trial of daily use of at least one dose a day.

COENZYME Q10, FROM SOYBEAN AND CORN OILS, A MIRACLE ANTI-AGING FOOD?

Coenzyme Q10 is one of the active ingredients in keeping your cells healthy. It works in helping to convert the food we eat into energy in the cell so that they can divide to make new cells, and to heal wounds. As we get older the cells operate less efficiently, and consequently we heal more slowly, and we even seem to have less energy. By using soybean and corn oil in our diet we can go a long ways toward keeping our cells healthy and active. Studies have shown that having adequate levels of Q10 in the diet result in both looking younger and feeling younger. There is not so much concern about minor injuries that did not bother us when we were younger, but which cause problems that take months to solve themselves when we are older. If you aren't using corn oil or soybean oil in your diet at this time you would be wise to start now. It doesn't have to be for every meal, but it should be every day.

STRENGTHEN THE GLAND THAT CONTROLS AGING THROUGH DIET

From the best information available it seems that the thymus gland controls much of our aging process. The thymus is very active when we are young, reaches a peak at around 20, and then declines to the point that it disappears in the aged. The thymus acts to manage our immune system, and the healthier the immune system, the healthier we are. It seems reasonable that if we can keep our thymus operating at a high level as we grow older we will stay healthier, and age more slowly. After all, the problem of getting older is not just that we want to live longer, but that we want to live healthier too.

The thymus has become much more familiar with the growth in AIDS and all of the talk about killer T-cells. These cells are very effective in countering infections and keeping us healthy. The source of T-cells is the thymus gland, and the 'T' in T-cell stands for thymus.

It is now well known why the thymus produces fewer and

fewer T-cells as we age, although the result is easy to see. The older we get the slower we tend to heal from cuts, bruises and breaks. We also get sicker, and develop disabilities from many diseases that bothered us little if at all when we were younger. The cause of many of these bad activities is thought to be closely related to the decline in thymus activity in producing T-cells.

While a decline in thymus function might be a normal process in getting older, we now know that we can reverse it to some degree, and stop much of the decline from happening at all. The thymus seems to be especially sensitive to the presence of trace elements in the diet. The best way to ensure adequate trace elements is to eat a varied diet with lots of whole grains and fruits, and stay off of diets that restrict you to just a few foods.

The trace elements most often mentioned are zinc, that promotes thymus activity, vitamin A, that prevents the thymus from declining in function, and vitamin E, that helps the thymus maintain a maximum productivity. Sources of these foods are pork and turkey, for zinc, in the meats. The best vegetable foods are spinach, brown rice, wheat, and yogurt. Whole wheat is also good for vitamin E, and vegetable oils are another excellent source of vitamin E. Vitamin A can be found in many vegetable foods. Some of the best are greens, carrots, spinach, sweet potatoes, and winter squash. The foods listed here are just meant to get you started. If you would like more complete lists consult any basic book on nutrition, but whatever you do note that whole wheat includes many of the vitamins and minerals that are listed as necessary to keep a healthy thymus, and a healthy immune system.

THE VITAMIN THAT COMBATS OXIDATION AT THE CELL LEVEL TO COUNTER AGING

Aging brings on a variety of diseases that are caused by oxidation. To counter this process, which occurs all of our lives but gets worse as we get older, we need to increase our intake of antioxidants at the same time. One of the best, and most effective antioxidants is vitamin E. Now before you say that you know everything you need to know about vitamin E let me run through some of the benefits, and then give you a list of some of the foods where you can get it naturally. Of course if you wish to take it in capsule form, and most people do, that is just fine, but many of us would prefer to use natural sources for our vitamins whenever we can.

The premier benefit of vitamin E is its effectiveness against cancer. It has long been known that vitamin E prevent cancer by decreasing the free radicals in our blood that we get from oxidation. Besides cancer, it also helps in healing wounds. It seems that as we get older our bodies heal less efficiently. Vitamin E will help to turn back the clock on healing from simple cuts and scrapes, but should also be used when you have surgery. The time it takes to heal after surgery can often be cut dramatically through the use of high doses of vitamin E. Of course with surgery you will also be taking other medications and you should ask your doctor even before taking vitamin E to make certain that you will not get any side effects from the combination of drugs you are taking and the vitamin E. Even if your doctor does want you to take internal doses you can still use it on the outside of your body if your surgery was external. Don't do anything that your doctor tells you will hurt you, but use vitamin E whenever you can in case of wounds or surgeries.

Now just so that I don't have to write a whole book about the uses of vitamin E I will just give a list of some of the other problems that it can be used to cure or prevent:

acne	arthritis	athlete's foot
boils	burns	bloodcirculation
cold sores	cracked skin	cysts
dandruff	eczema	fingernails
gum problems	heart disease	herpes type II
high blood pressure	itching	leg cramps
leg pain	leg ulcers	leukoplakia
menopause problem	muscle pain	phlebitis
psoriasis	ringworm	scar tissue
shingles	sinus problems	

Now if you are sold on the need for vitamin E in your diet, and this can be true as much for problems in the young as in the old, I will give you a few of the foods that you should eat daily. The food sources commonly listed are wheat germ, whole grains, and vegetable oils. Wheat germ is found in whole wheat, but it is hard to get a sufficient dose of vitamin E by eating whole wheat. Most people use vitamin E in a powdered form that they put on top of their morning cereal or add to the foods they eat. However, I prefer the natural sources and always use vegetable oils at home, and only use whole grain breads and cereals. If you combine these three sources of vitamin E, and eat them through the day, you should be able to keep the level in your body high and constant. Oh yes, one other drawback that I have depending entirely upon wheat germ is that I find it a little bitter on my cereal or in drinks. When you use whole grains and vegetable oils you can combine the wheat germ sources with other foods to get a much larger variety. After all, it is the daily use of vitamin E that does you good, not just taking it for a few months and getting sick of the source. I will leave it up to you to decide on your best source, but whatever you decide I would make a definite effort to put vitamin E into your daily diet.

A TEA TO HELP YOU FEEL AND LOOK YOUNGER

The oldest teas written into history are from the Chinese. These teas go back for at least 5000 years, and include every medical problem known to man. It is not unexpected that they also include teas to counter the effects of aging which will help you to feel and look younger. The only problem is finding one of these teas among all of the thousands of teas that the Chinese offer. By great good luck I have found a formula for one which is very popular with the Chinese, and which you can make with ingredients from a health food store, your garden, or a Chinese pharmacy. You can even have a Chinese native druggist make up a tea mix if you can't find one already made up, or if you don't want to do it yourself. To get this done all that you have to do is go into a Chinese pharmacy with a list of the ingredients, and the amounts of each, and they will make it up for you. I am going to give you that list, and then you can decide how you would like to go about getting it made up.

The Chinese call their teas for the aged long life tea, and they have several different kinds. Each kind varies according to the needs of the patient. That is whether or not they are healthy, the type of illness they have if they are not healthy, and the time of year in which it is taken. This makes a lot of sense since some ingredients are probably more potent at some times of the year than at others, and not everyone needs the same medicines no matter how old they they are. The ingredients for the first tea are for people who are weak and tend to be cold. The tea is called Cinnamon Herb Tea, or Kuei Chih Tang:

Cinnamon -- 4 grams

Ginger ------ 4 grams

Peony alba - 5 grams

Jujube ------- 4 grams

Licorice ----- 4 grams

For illnesses like colds and congestion the Chinese offer Ephedra Herb Tea, or Mao Huang Tang, which is composed of:

Ephedra ---------- 5 grams

Apricot kernal -- 5 grams

Cinnamon ------- 4 grams

Licorice -------- 1.5 grams

For those with a combination of cold and flu symptoms which also include stiffness, chills, perspiration and fever, the Chinese offer Pueraria Tea, also called Ko Ken Tang, which is composed of:

Pueraria ----- 6 grams	Jujube --------- 4 grams
Peony alba -- 4 grams	Cinnamon ---- 4 grams
Ginger -------- 4 grams	
Licorice ----- 1.5 grams	

For the best effects these Chinese teas should be prepared as what is called a decoction. That is, the ingredients should be placed in a pan and gently boiled for up to one hour, at which time about half of the water should be evaporated. If you are able to find a company selling a granular form of the teas, in which the active ingredients have already been extracted, they may be prepared simply in hot water, and consumed as you would an English tea. In either case they should be used daily for best effect, and several times a day is much better than using them only once a day.

ALLERGIES

Allergies are miserable problems for many people, and allergies can be caused by just about anything. One of the things that makes allergies so frustrating is that you never know when you are going to get an attack, and most of the time you don't even know what you are allergic to. Most often allergy attacks are mistaken for summer colds, but that is only because you usually get a runny nose and sneeze a lot. But some allergies are serious and can make you stay indoors for weeks at a time. Personally I defy allergies, but I can only do that because I don't have any severe allergies. For a friend of mine with asthma allergy attacks can also bring on asthma attacks which are much more serious. Asthma can even be life threatening in some people, and anyone with the problem should not fool around with allergies when they can avoid them.

Avoiding allergies is more easily said than done. Since the substances we are allergic to travel in the air as well as the dust of our homes and streets, just living will usually result in your exposure to substances to which you are allergic. This is where the use of allergy alleviating foods comes in. With a diet that helps you to avoid allergy attacks you can carry out a normal life without worrying every day if you are going to end up looking like a snivelling, sneezing, runny eyed, pathetic, beggar instead of the forceful and competent person that you really are.

FOODS THAT CAN END ALLERGY MISERY

I can offer a couple of suggestions that can either relieve or alleviate allergy attacks. Of course there is a difference between preventing allergies from bothering you, and curing their effects after you have developed an attack. In case of allergy attacks prevention will usually lead to a quick stoppage of symptoms since allergies are not infections, and once you prevent the allergic substance from affecting you your symptoms will clear up rapidly.

First I would like you to try a nice herbal tea called chamomile. Chamomile contains a substance called azulene, which has been shown to prevent allergic seizures in animals. Chamomile has been used as a folk remedy against allergies for many years, and can be taken as a tea or inhaled in vapor form. Chamomile is accepted by the medical community, and a chamomile throat spray is sold in health food stores which is used to treat asthma attacks. It seems to work by keeping the air ways open, and preventing them from closing up when they come in contact with allergic substances.

Another remedy with a long history is watercress. Watercress can be purchased in the super market, and eaten raw by the handful as well as in salads and sandwiches. It is most effective in relieving watery eyes, sneezing, and stuffiness in the head.

For milk lovers there are milk products containing lactobacillus acidophilus, which is available in some milk as an additive, and which can be found in all yogurt. You have probably been told to eat yogurt after developing diarrhea in order to get the right kind of bacteria in your digestive system, and this is good advice. In fact you should eat yogurt every day during the allergy season to help prevent allergy attacks in the first place. Allergies should not be feared, at least not while you can take steps to prevent ever getting allergy attacks. The recommendations given here are just a few of the many you might use, and these can be picked up at your local market for a very reasonable price.

ALZHEIMER'S

Alzheimer's is a disease that causes what we used to call senility, and which we used to think was part of the natural process of aging. We now know that the symptoms of senility are not a natural process of anything, but are caused by diseases which can be treated, even if we do not yet know how to cure them. The picture we get of a senile person is someone who is forgetful of himself, his friends, and even his family, and who becomes less and less able to take care of himself. These senile old people gradually draw into themselves until in their last years they simply exist, apparently uncomprehending of the rest of the world, until they pass on.

However, since much of this senility is known to be caused by Alzheimer's disease, and its effects on the chemical processes of the brain, we can treat it to some degree with diet and drugs to prevent some of the symptoms even if we can't stop the disease completely.

ALZHEIMER'S CAN BE PREVENTED WITH THE RIGHT FOODS

Alzheimer's is strongly associated with the buildup of aluminum in the body. By avoiding foods with aluminum, so the thinking goes, you can also prevent the development of Alzheimer's. The logic of these seems to make a lot of sense, and it is certainly worth considering. We get a lot of aluminum in our diet from our cooking utensils, particularly when we cook with aluminum pots. The foods which contribute the most aluminum to our diet when cooked in these pots are those that are acidic. Acidic foods include tomatoes, fruits, and cabbage. For those of you who like to prepare their own spaghetti sauce, you should never do it in an aluminum pot since the tomatoes in the sauce will result in a high level of aluminum in your spaghetti sauce. A few years ago aluminum mugs were popular, and were especially good for drinking wine. If you have any of these old mugs around never use them for wine, tomato juice, or any fruit juices. Aluminum coffee pots were also used a lot in the past and can be easily found in many homes and garage sales today. If you have one get rid of it, and if you don't, then don't buy one. Coffee is highly acidic and you are getting a much more potent dose of aluminum in your coffee than you are getting of caffeine.

Other foods to avoid, and of course how much you have used them depends on your own diet habits, include processed cheeses, nondairy creamers, self-rising flour and cake mixes, and buffered aspirin. You need to find substitutes for each one of these, or simply cut out their use altogether.

Should you doubt that these steps are necessary you should know that aluminum migrates through the body and gathers around the nerve spindles which control memory and muscle control, and it is found in high concentrations in the brain of all Alzheimer's patients. It is also true that most of the aluminum that comes into your body through food simply passes through the digestive tract without being absorbed, but the amount that is absorbed can do a lot of damage. It is even possible that at some point, after years of repeated attacks from aluminum, the nerves begin to deteriorate on the way to developing Alzheimer's. This may mean that you can prevent it from happening to you by limiting, or eliminating aluminum from your diet and your medicine cabinet.

2 FOODS THAT CAN HELP PREVENT YOU FROM GETTING ALZHEIMER'S DISEASE

I could give you a long list of foods that don't contain aluminum, and tell you that by eating them you could prevent Alzheimer's, but that wouldn't help you at all if you were already committed to an aluminum containing food and didn't even know it. No, what you need are foods that will protect you from the small amount of aluminum you are going to have in your diet no matter how careful you try to be, and even if you have a meal occasionally that is very high in aluminum. There are two strategies for preventing Alzheimer's by minimizing the damage that aluminum can do to you. You can prevent it from acting at all, and best recommended for that is choline, or you can minimize its accumulation in the brain by using foods high in calcium.

There are many foods which are good sources of choline, but the one which is my best choice is brown rice. A 4 once serving of brown rice contains 650 milligrams of choline, and you should be able to mix 4 ounces into your diet pretty much every day since that is only a few spoonfuls. While brown rice is what I prefer egg yolks are much higher in choline, though of course they also have saturated fats, and liver or caviar have about the same amount of choline, but I eat liver only once every couple of months, and caviar about once every couple of years. You need a good source that you can eat nearly every day to keep the nerves in your brain sharp and the affects from aluminum attacks at a minimum.

On the calcium side most people think first of milk and cheese or cottage cheese.   While these are some of the best sources of calcium in our diet I am bothered somewhat by the amount of fat that you can get in all of them if you use the most common forms. Luckily all of these come in low fat and fat free types, and I would advise you to use one of those. Oh, and the choice I recommend above the others is milk. Not everyone wants to eat cheese every day, and anyone who tries to eat cottage cheese every day will get sick of it eventually, but most of us can drink milk in some form or other several times a day and feel perfectly happy about it.

AN AMINO ACID TO HELP RESTORE MENTAL SHARPNESS AND MEMORY

Amino acids make up the proteins that we get in meats and whole grain cereals. There are a total of 8 of these in a complete protein, such as you find in eggs, and they work to build every part of the body and keep it healthy. But one, taurine, is especially important in brain function. When taurine levels fall epileptics have more seizures, and even infants seem to have more problems. Taurine is especially active in the brain, as well as being one of the most abundant amino acids in the body.

The question is what should you do to keep your taurine levels high, or to bring them up if you think that they are low? Of course you can take supplements of taurine, which you can get from a health food store or a pharmacy, but there are also many natural sources that are cheaper and that you should have anyway. Whole grain cereals such as wheat are excellent sources. But so are eggs, milk, and red meats.

Unless you are on a restricted diet of some kind you should have no trouble getting sufficient taurine in your diet, but if you are sick, have had an operation, or have undergone a stress in your life you may need to increase your level of taurine for a time. All of these events result in depressed levels of taurine, and often result in a loss of appetite which just compounds the problem.

People react differently to stress. Some stop eating altogether for days, mope around their homes, and constantly feel deep depression. While mourning a loss or feeling sorry over a mistake is natural, it does not mean that someone has to also be depressed for the entire mourning period, which can take a year or more. At this time you let your memory wander and all that it seems to do is take you deeper into depression and make you less able to cope with the needs of everyday life. Don't do that to yourself.

You need to take a proactive role in your health, and making sure that your diet has adequate levels of the nutrients you need, such as taurine, is one of the first steps you should take. Have a steak, or a couple of pieces of whole wheat toast, or even just a yogurt. It may not solve all of your problems, but at least it will help to keep you sharp enough to deal with your own needs.

ANEMIA

Anemia is a failure by the body to make enough red blood cells, and it can be caused by either disease or diet. Avoiding anemia, when we are otherwise healthy, requires a diet with enough proteins and iron to build the red blood cells that carry oxygen around in the body. Not taking care of anemia puts us at risk for damage to all of the cells in our body, and even to heart attacks and strokes from the lack of necessary oxygen that they need. Since this is a book about diet I will offer some ideas , what you can do in your diet to heal and control anemia ,should you get it. Only a doctor can diagnose anemia accurately, and only a doctor can tell you exactly why you have it. But this shouldn't prevent you from taking any precautions that you can that might prevent it from occurring, or even cure the condition in some cases.

IT CAN BE HEALED WITH THE RIGHT DIET

There are three kinds of anemia so I will offer three types of diet that can help. The first, and most common, is iron deficiency anemia, the second is pernicious anemia, and the third is megaloblastic anemia. A different diet is required for each type, and the more you know about your diet needs the better. Again, don't depend on your own judgements as to the cause of your anemia, get a diagnosis from a doctor before making any decisions as to what to do about it with diet or anything else.

Iron deficiency anemia you had best attack it in terms of the deficiency that is most likely to be the cause, a shortage of iron in the diet. As I mentioned above, we get a lot of iron in red meat, but even so some forms of dietary iron are more easily used by the body than others. Meat, fish, and poultry have the highest levels, and eggs, beans, nuts, and whole grains are second best. Do not depend upon spinach as a source of iron since only a very small amount of its iron can be used by the body.

Pernicious anemia is caused by an entirely different problem, a deficiency of B-12 in the diet. It is much more rare than iron deficiency anemia, but the symptoms are pretty much identical. The best sources of B-12 are eggs, meat, milk, and cheese. By looking above it is easy to see that these are also recommended foods for iron deficiency anemia. Thus if you have an anemia problem you can use the same diet for a cure whether it is iron deficiency anemia or pernicious anemia. If you have a medical problem that prevents you from absorbing B-12 that is in your diet you may have to resort to B-12 shots. While a doctor will give these shots, you can be instructed on how to do it for yourself or to have a friend or family member do it in order to save most of the cost.

Megaloblastic anemia is caused by another type of deficiency, folic acid. Symptoms of fatigue and exhaustion are common to all anemia, but in addition you will suffer a decreased interest in sex, gastrointestinal discomfort, and a sore and shiny tongue among other things. Vegetarians rarely suffer from this form of anemia since the best sources of folic acid are green leafy vegetables.

This goes for everyone, if you have any kind of a regular problem with fatigue and exhaustion, whatever the other symptoms, you should check your diet first. See that you have green leafy vegetables in your daily diet, but also that you include whole grains, meat, cheese, and eggs. At least two servings of these each day as well as two of green leafy vegetables. It doesn't matter whether you eat meat or not, the key is eating a wide variety of foods in your daily diet if you wish to prevent the development of a deficiency disease. Never accept a diet based on a single, or very limited, food source no matter how well the argument is put to you. No diet that is too narrow will give your body all of the nutrients it needs to stay healthy.

ANGINA CHEST PAIN

Angina means heart pain. The more complete term you might hear from your doctor is angina pectorus, which is chest pain. It is a sign of heart disease, and is the result of the heart being starved for blood carrying oxygen. The most common treatment is the use of nitro-glycerin tablets which open the arteries and let more blood pass through the heart. Untreated angina will result in a heart attack in the end, and will leave the victim in pain every time he exerts himself a little bit. In fact the chest pain is a sign that you have exerted yourself, and it lets you know that your heart isn't getting all of the nutrients that it needs.

FOODS THAT ALLEVIATE THIS EXCRUCIATING PAIN

From Chinese medicine we learn that both hawthorne and chrysanthemum teas have been used as treatments for angina. If you have experienced angina attacks a good preventive measure might be to include the use of one or both of these teas in your regular diet. To make chrysanthemum tea you can get the tea directly from a health food store, or you can grow it yourself in your own garden. To make it directly from the plant cut 6 tablespoons of flowers, and divide them into 4 equal portions. This will be a one day supply. To make the tea boil water and pour it directly over one portion of the flowers and let steep for about 15 minutes. You can then remove the flowers and sweeten if necessary, or drink directly. Have your first tea when you get up, and then the other portions at about 4 hour intervals. Repeat this procedure every day for at least a month. Tests have found 80% to 90% of angina patients to be helped with the use of this tea, and blood pressure usually returns to normal within about a week.

Hawthorne can be taken in two forms, either as a capsule or a tea. Hawthorne capsules are sold in health food stores, and are made by Nature's Way. About 2 to 3 capsules a day are recommended for relief of angina. The tea is made directly from hawthorne berries. Enough berries should be crushed so that 1 1/2 tablespoons can be used in the preparation. First soak the crushed berries for 8 hours in 2 cups of cold water. At the end of the 8 hours bring the berries and water to a boil and remove from the stove. Strain the mixture, and sweeten the tea as desired.

If you are not using capsules the chrysanthemum tea is much easier to prepare than the hawthorne tea. Nevertheless I have given both since one may work better for one person than another. It is also of interest that hawthorne has been recommended for a wider range of circulatory disorders and heart problems.

A word of warning is always in order when discussing problems of the heart and blood circulation. Because of the capacity of these illnesses to kill and cause serious disability you should always be diagnosed by a physician if you suspect such a problem. If you do not have a doctor that you trust, and you do not wish to put your health into the hands of regular Western doctors, you may be a good candidate for a holistic physician. Such doctors are still licensed physicians, but they are more widely trained and should also be aware of diet therapies as well as Western chemical methods of treatment. With a little looking you can find one, and you may just decide that you like the care they give you better than what you had experienced in the past.

ARTHRITIS

Arthritis is any painful swelling of any joint in the body. We can get it in our fingers, shoulders, elbows, neck, ankles, or anywhere else that our bones come together. There are also many causes, and most of the time the causes can't be cured, but they can almost always be relieved. In fact for most forms of arthritis relief amounts to a cure, if only for a day. When an attack is brought on by muscle strain treating the joint so that the pain and swelling go away, along with a little rest, will result in a complete cure. But if the arthritis is brought on by some sort of growth around a joint, or deterioration of the joint from an injury, the best we can hope for is relief that will last through the day. Not surprisingly this last kind is what we tend most to get as we grow older. It may be of comfort to know that by the age of 30 everyone has had an episode of arthritis, although the causes are often unique. What is also important is that you can take dietary precautions against getting arthritis, as well as use diet to cure yourself of attacks when they do occur. I will begin by offering you 2 foods that will help you prevent getting arthritis in the first place.

WHAT YOU ARE LACKING

Because arthritis is a disease of the joints, much dietary attention has been paid to what nutritional elements are required for healthy joint fluid. This fluid is called synovial fluid, and it is something that is not found in any other part of the body. The purpose of synovial fluid is to lubricate the joints moving against each other, in the same way that oil lubricates a car engine to keep it running smoothly. When the snyovial fluid isn't doing its job, no matter what the reason, the joints will rub against each other when they move and the whole area will get sore and swollen. This is a pretty fair description of what arthritis looks like and feels like.

By this approach, any time that you are getting arthritic pain it is an indication that your synovial fluid isn't doing its job. Getting the fluid the nutrition it needs is the first step to preventing arthritic attacks. Studies of synovial fluid of people who have arthritis has found low levels of vitamin C, folic acid, zinc, pantothenic acid, and vitamin D.

While foods should be the main source of your nutrients, I would also recommend that you add a good multi-vitamin to your diet if you have encountered arthritis pain. While this is not the ideal solution, it does provide a short term solution that you can follow while you are working out an ideal diet high in all of these nutrients, and appropriate to your own tastes.

TWO FOODS THAT CAN HELP PREVENT ARTHRITIS

Dietary treatments are based on the idea that arthritis is an auto-immune disease, in which your body is attacking itself, and that arthritis sufferers have deficiencies of such vitamins as C, D, and B-complex. While these are two separate ideas on the main causes, and would require different types of treatments, oddly they end up recommending the same foods for prevention and treatment. what this means to me is that the foods have long been known to be effective for arthritis, and that the various doctors who have been studying it have looked for ways to account for the cures that they already know exist.

The first preventive is fish. By one theory fish is supposed to cure the auto-immune cause of arthritis since it contains omega-3 fatty acids. Of course it also contains a lot of other minerals and vitamins as well, and this may be why the vitamin deficiency people also recommend it. If for some reason you do not wish to eat fish you can take fish oil capsules and get the same effects. Many of the best features of fish are also found in cod liver oil, and that can also be taken in capsules. Many Americans not eating fish might be one of the reasons that we have so much arthritis in the country in the first place.

To go more over to the other side you should also use whole grains as an arthritis preventor. Whole grain wheat may be the best, put whole grains into your diet now, if they aren't already. Whole grain wheat is particularly good as a source of B-vitamins. Many older people stop eating whole grains because they develop problems in their digestion, but cutting out the whole grains, along with the fruits and vegetables, probably cause a lot more problems than it cures. You should have 3 or 4 servings daily of whole grain, whether as bread or cereal. Whole grains not only give you a wide range of vitamins, but they also help to keep your digestion regular by putting roughage into your diet.

FOODS THAT CAN BRING RELIEF WHEN IT HURTS

While it's true that foods can bring relief to arthritic pains, you don't eat them to get the relief. Foods act by changing your body chemistry, that is by preventing your body from developing the arthritic condition in the first place. However, if you are hav-ing an arthritic attack what you need is relief right now. The quickest way to get that is through the use of a poultice. Even doctors recommend the use of heat on arthritic joints, but the use of a poultice is one step better since your body can absorb some medicinal elements through the skin in the same way that they can through shots or when you eat them. With this in mind I will give you a couple of recommendations for poultices that have proved very effective in getting quick relief from the arthritic joint pain.

The first of these is something that you can get from your supermarket, and something that you should have in your diet anyway. Go to the market and buy some fresh cabbage. Peal off 6 complete leaves, and cut out the midribs (that is the large ribs in the middle of the leaves). Then take an iron and apply heat to the leaves until they soften up and they feel like a piece of cloth. Now put a little vegetable oil on your skin, place the leave over the sore joint, or joints, in overlapping layers, and cover everything with a towel. If there is no relief within an hour repeat the process with fresh, warm, cabbage leaves. This procedure works for instant relief of arthritis pain. It is not surprising that cabbage should work for arthritis since it is also recommended for cancer prevention, to fight yeast infections, and to heal ulcers.

Another food remedy from the supermarket is figs. Figs are always dried, but that is okay. Take 6 figs and put them into 3 cups of boiling water. Leave in the water until they soften up, and then mash them. Take the fresh. warm, fig mash and cover the sore joint with it, covering the fig poultice with a towel or heavy cloth. This should remain on the sore spot for 1/2 an hour at least, and if you can cover it with a heating pad it can be used for a couple of hours. Besides its use as a poultice for sore joints figs are also effective as cancer preventives, and as a natural laxative when taken internally.

FOODS CAN MAKE YOU THINK YOU HAVE IT WHEN YOU DON'T, HOW TO KNOW

Arthritis has many causes, and some of these causes are allergies to the foods we eat. It has long been known that high cholesterol foods are associated with arthritis, but the whole family of nightshade plants are also a common cause. Certainly anyone with arthritis should make certain that their cholesterol levels are as low as possible, and they should also take account of how many nightshade plants they have in their diets.

Cholesterol is found most consistently in red meats, but also in egg yolks. If you don't want to become a vegetarian, and it is perfectly all right if you do, then you need to go to foods such as fish to avoid cholesterol. While it is not a favorite of very many people, sardines are an excellent source of non-red meat protein that counteracts arthritis.

On the other hand we have many nightshade plants in our diets, and most of the time we are not even aware that we are eating them. One of the most common is potatoes. There is always a little debate going on as to whether you should eat potatoes that have re-greened, that is where the potatoes have gotten green after you have stored them for a while. The debate is based on the danger of nightshade, and that the toxins are found in the green portion of the plants.

The list of common dietary nightshade plants includes tomatoes, potatoes, eggplant, and peppers. Eggplant and peppers do not usually make up much of anyone's diet, but potatoes and tomatoes can make up the major portion of many diets. But since these are such a big part of so many diets it is important to know if they are really dangerous before everyone stops eating them.

The scientific way of doing this, and you can do it yourself, is to begin by cutting all nightshade foods out of your diet. Do not concern yourself if you are having or not having arthritic attacks at this time since other factors may be the cause. Once you have a nightshade free diet, stay on it for one full week. Then one at a time introduce the nightshade foods into your diet that you were using before, and watch for arthritis symptoms. You can be pretty certain that your arthritis is caused, at least partly, by nightshade family foods.

ARTERIES CLOSING UP?

Clogged arteries are not something that happens overnight. In fact it is something that takes most of our lives to become critical, but once it gets to that point it can result in heart attacks and strokes. The usual culprits are saturated fats and cholesterol, which is not too unusual since the American diet often contains too much of both of these. The good news is that just because you have been eating poorly for many years it doesn't mean that you have to have a stroke or heart attack. With the proper foods you can counter the effects of your poor diet habits, and even reverse the processes through which your arteries were getting clogged.

FOODS THAT CAN HELP TO OPEN THEM AGAIN

Looking for foods that open clogged arteries leads back to the whole grains again. We have encountered whole grains before in many areas, but they are also very useful for removing fat deposits from the arteries. We have seen that wheat has many uses, and this is another one. Others, which have an even greater following are rye, barley, and oats. A few years ago oats were widely talked about as protective against cancer as well, and even though the talk has quieted down oats still have a great number of uses.

The preparation of these whole grains is really very simple: they are available as cooked breakfast cereals, in breads, some of them in cold breakfast cereals, and even in some baked goods such as muffins. I would not advise using the baked goods as first choices though since they also contain a lot of fat that you don't need no matter what other problems you may have. The best choices are the breakfast cereals and breads. With the popularity of fat free foods these days you can probably even find a low fat or fat free bread made with whole grains. They will be harder and drier than the other types, but they will be much better for you over the long run.

There is one other method for removing clogs from the arteries, short of surgery, and it is called chelation. This procedure is done in the hospital, and uses a medication called EDTA. In this procedure the EDTA is dripped into your blood stream over a period of time and dissolves the blockages in the arteries. It is very expensive, as compared to dietary solutions, but it may work where diet doesn't. Since no cure can be guaranteed, chelation should be considered along with surgery when natural cures don't. It is good to know though that often times natural treatments work when medical ones don't. But no doctor is going to give credit to a dietary cure for a disease or illness that he is treating unsuccessfully with all of his medical skills. He does want to be paid doesn't he?

BACK PAIN

Back pain can have many causes. Stress can cause back pain as well as pain in many other parts of the body. Injury is always a possibility, and collapsed or ruptured discs are the most common cause. Among the causes must certainly be included strain of the lower back, such as you can get with poor lifting techniques, or which some people get just getting up wrong or twisting in the wrong direction. Deterioration of the spinal column due to injury or disease is probably the most serious, but is also the least common. No matter what the cause the result will be inflammation and pain in the lower back.

If you have never had lower back pain than you do not have a clear idea of the disability that it can cause. Lower back pain prevents you from bending over normally, from getting dressed even when sitting on the edge of your bed, and can cause you great pain when driving. When the pain is severe you can't do anything except try to find a way to sit or lie that relieves some of the pain.

The importance of this problem, which most of us will be visited by one or more times in our lives, is such that solutions are needed. Doctors often recommend a warm compress or hot water bottle to the lower back to relax the muscles and promote blood flow. I certainly support that although I think it is best that the compress be combined with a poultice that helps to hold the heat and can even add some healing ingredients.

We have already touched upon this in relation to arthritis pain, and it works just as well with lower back pain--so just try a cabbage poultice to your lower back. Chinese medicine also has a couple of good teas for lower back pain, but you will be best off going to a Chinese medical practitioner to get them since they are made with plants and herbs that you can't buy at your local market.

If you have exhausted all of the herbal and natural remedies, and you still have back pain, you may now be considering surgery. I will tell you that you are just as likely to get more back pain from surgery as less. In fact the surgeons who do these operations never guarantee that you will be pain free, even if the operations are considered a success, and of course you pay the bill no matter how the operation comes out.

One alternative to surgery which you can do if natural remedies haven't worked is injection of chymopapain. This enzyme is derived from papayas, and has to be administered by a doctor. This is definitely not something that should be taken lightly, but it also doesn't require that you be entered into a hospital to get it.

The chymopapain is derived from ripe papayas and is then injected into low back pain sufferers under a light general anesthetic. It is injected directly into the disc that is causing the trouble, and fluoroscopy is used to help guide the injection. While this therapy has been effective in about 80% of the patients who have used it, there are side effects. The worst of the side effects is an inflammation of the spinal cord which can result in some paralysis and shock. These side effects are probably the result of the needle rather than the chymopapain that is injected, but they can't be avoided. However, because of the side effects most doctors have stopped using this type of therapy. Back surgery for pain requires about one year for recovery, and often results in no relief or a worsening of symptoms. While it does help many patients I feel that the risks are at least as great as the benefits, and that surgery should only be used as an absolute last resort.

BLINDNESS

Blindness is frightening to many people even though there is a large population of blind people in the United States. Most of those who are blind are older Americans, but it can happen to anyone by accident. In some countries blindness is much more common since they have diseases that affect children and adults along with the aged. Luckily we do not have any of those particular diseases here to deal with. What we do have is a problem of progressive loss of sight with age to the point that many people in their later years are unable to drive, read, or even watch television. While this is a common problem in the aged, it is not inevitable. It is possible to prevent blindness in many cases, or at least to delay the development of blindness in those who have already developed problems that may lead to blindness eventually.

FOODS THAT CAN PREVENT AND FIGHT-OFF AGE RELATED BLINDNESS

One of the early signs of blindness, and one that you should never ignore, is night blindness. Night blindness is dangerous all by itself, since it can result in traffic accidents, and it often leads to serious eye disease and total blindness. Now the good thing about night blindness is that it can often be treated with vitamin A. Long term vitamin A deficiency is a frequent cause, and increasing your intake of foods like carrots, yams, squash, and broccoli will bring your vitamin A levels up.

A shortage of vitamin B-2 will also affect the eyes, leaving them feeling itchy, burning, and watering. Vitamin B-2 is necessary for proper oxygenation of the eyes, so that when it is too low the blood vessels will attempt to carry more blood into the area resulting in all of the symptoms. Some good choices for B-2 are liver, chicken, egg yolk, and wheat germ. If you have any kind of regular eye discomfort you should check your levels of vitamin B-2 foods.

BLOOD FAT LEVELS

Everyone has fat in their blood. That is perfectly natural and normal, but it is the type of fat that you have to look at in addition to the amount that you have. High levels of fat in blood-are found in people who have a lot of fat in their diets. There are two important facts to keep in mind when you are considering blood fat levels and their relationship to diet. The first is that you should have as little fat in your diet as possible, these days no more than 20 to 50 milligrams per day is recommended. As a comparison the normal American diet contains over 150 milligrams--is that a clue as to why we have so much arterial blockage leading to heart attacks and strokes. The other factor of great importance is that the fat you do get should be poly unsaturated. In general saturated fats are found in red meat, although they are also in avocados, and unsaturated fats are found in vegetables. The ratio of saturated to unsaturated fats is the way that blood fat levels are evaluated to see if you have a good diet or a dangerous diet. In any case I would like to offer you a few suggestions as to how blood fat levels can be controlled.

HOW THEY CAN BE CONTROLLED

There are several diets and dietary changes you can make that can help you lower your blood fat levels. The standard diet recommended by doctors consists of the use of polyunsaturated vegetable oils for frying and baking, increasing the amount of fish you eat and decreasing red meat, and decreasing your use of eggs and dairy products. This diet works quite well in lowering blood fat levels and increasing the P/S ratio. But there are other ways, and I want to give you some alternatives.

For those of you so inclined giving up meat altogether and going to a vegetarian diet will accomplish the same thing. Vegetarian diets naturally replace the saturated fats with unsaturated fats since those are the types of fat found in vegetable foods. Furthermore if you eat a well balanced diet of fruits and vegetables you will not have a protein problem, you will probably lose weight over time, and your blood pressure will drop.

BLOOD PRESSURE

Maintaining normal blood pressure is essential to keeping disease free. More people die from blood pressure problems than from any other cause, and most of the time they don't even know why they have the problem. Low blood pressure is a problem for some people, but high blood pressure is something nearly every one will have to face if they live long enough. It is said that part of the natural aging process is a rise in the blood pressure, but not every one has high blood pressure as they get older. In fact, even though doctors cannot account for 90% of the high blood pressure that we have, it is probably related to our diets and our life styles.

Look at all of the risk factors that are listed in the news-paper every time they talk about someone dying of a heart attack or a stroke: smoking is usually number one, being overweight is number two, then comes lack of exercise, high fat diets, and hardening of the arteries. But even given all of these there are choices you can make in your diet that will help you to keep your blood pressure where it belongs. By the way, normal pressure is listed as 120/80, if you see it on your doctor's chart. If your blood pressure gets down to 110/70 you have low blood pres-sure, and you have borderline high blood pressure if it goes to 140/100. At this level most doctors will want to put you on med-ication to lower your blood pressure, though I think that you still have a choice, and that you should make it. At 160/120 you are classed as have high blood pressure and doctor's will start dis-cussing the probability of a stroke or heart attack if you don't get it down with medication.   Of course our concern here is not to find a good medication for high blood pressure, but to find a diet that will help you to lower your blood pressure and avoid med-ications.

FOODS TO KEEP YOUR BLOOD PRESSURE WHERE IT BELONGS

Foods that will help you keep your blood pressure in the normal range fall into two categories. The first is foods to avoid that tend to raise your blood pressure, and the second is foods you can use to protect you from getting high blood pressure in the first place even if some of your diet isn't perfect.

Foods to avoid consist of red meats and all high fat foods, salt, and alcohol. There are other villains, but these are the big three that tend to drive your blood pressure up over the years. Fat, particularly saturated fat, does its dirty work by adding to the problem of hardening of the arteries. As the arter-ies narrow with deposits of fat it takes more energy from the heart to push the blood through your body. It's also just like pinching off a garden hose, the smaller you make the space for the water to go through the higher the pressure at that point and the farther the water squirts on the other side. The result, when this happens in the blood vessel is high blood pressure.

Salt has the same effect, but from a different direction. Salt dissolves in water, and blood is mostly water. When salt dissolves in it the water is changed so that it stays in the blood vessels longer, and the blood pressure goes up. The more salt that you have in your diet the more likely you will be to have an elevated blood pressure. Since the diseases of high blood pressure will happen without regard for the cause of the high blood pressure, you can get strokes and heart attacks just from having too much salt in your diet. However, if you put yourself on a low salt diet you will also have an almost immediate drop in pressure since your body will eliminate all of the extra salt within a few days.

Alcohol is a little different in its damage to your blood pressure system. Alcohol adds calories and weight to the body, which in turn cause high blood pressure. But alcohol is also a muscle toxin that interferes with the function of the body such that it could trigger a heart attack or stroke by minor changes in the function of the heart, or of some other muscle groups in the body. Alcohol may not carry the same risk as some of the other factors, but there is a definite risk to drinking when you have a blood pressure problem.

Now I have promised to give you some foods that can protect you even if you don't have the best possible diet. A nice little alphabetical list of some of the most common foods you can use for your blood pressure are:

asparagus	bananas
beans	celery
garlic	onions
mango	tomatoes

The ways in which these foods protect you from high

blood pressure differ greatly, but can be summed up to say that they range from eliminating water from the blood, as in asparagus, to discouraging the clots that cause heart attacks and strokes, as in garlic and onions, to being a calmative of the heart muscle to keep it beating calmly, as with mango and bananas, and finally to providing high levels of potassium, as with bananas, beans, and tomatoes. All of these effects help the blood pressure to stay at its proper level. It is best that you use these foods in combination for the best overall effect. While food is food, it's obvious that some foods are more equal than others when it comes to helping us stay healthy.

BODY ACHE

Some people have body ache every day, and take pain killers to feel better. Others only hurt occasionally, and only in certain parts of their bodies. They may take pain killers and they may just get a rub down. Body ache, in its many forms, can be caused by disease, stress, arthritis, muscle strain, or toxins in our food. It is this last category we want to look at so far as causes, but it is all that we wish to view for prevention and cure.

CAN YOUR DIET CAUSE IT, PREVENT IT, OR RELIEVE IT?

Diet can cause body ache in a couple of obvious ways, if you eat too much you may very well develop body ache, and if you eat something toxic you will probably develop body ache. When any toxic substance attacks the muscles they respond by giving you pain. But not all toxic foods are toxic to the same people. An allergy can result in pain, but more likely you have a food item that has been contaminated with a poison. Either one that has grown on it or one that has been spilled on it. These types of pain should be controlled at the source since you cannot prevent the pain once you have been poisoned. Still, pain from part of your diet is going to be one of the minor sources, and even if you prevent all attacks of body ache from your diet you will not cut out more than 5% of the pain attacks you will experience.

Diet is also not much of a preventive of body ache. Since you don't know the source in advance, and it will probably be related to a disease like the flu, it is only by avoiding the flu that you can avoid the body ache that accompanies it. The same goes pretty much for all food preventives of body ache. Don't eat foods you are allergic to. Don't eat foods that have spoiled so that you get poisoned. Otherwise just don't overeat, and don't drink so much of any thing that you feel sick.

Diet for a cure of your body ache has a little more promise, since there is a substance that relieves body ache and you can get it in food. The actual natural pain reliever is manufactured in the brain. The name of it is endorphins, and the ways that it is released are several. Studies have found increased endorphins in the blood following acupuncture treatments, and the taking of placebos. Placebos are used in medicine to test the effectiveness of new medications, and if a medicine is no better than a placebo in relieving symptoms it is concluded that the medicine is ineffective. Considering placebos as promoters of endorphin release a medicine that relieves symptoms as well as a placebo might be a perfectly good medicine, and if it does better it could be the result of having some medicinal effect in addition to the placebo effect.

In relation to diet though some foods also promote the release of these natural pain relievers, and can relieve body ache just as efficiently as any medical treatment. Compulsive eaters relieve the pain of the tensions they feel by eating. Compulsive shoppers, drinkers, and gamblers do the same thing. When you have body ache having a reasonable serving of your favorite food will help promote the release of endorphins, stimulating your pleasure center in the brain, and relieving your body ache. While this isn't a particular food it is certainly an effective pain relief strategy.

Endorphins are the last chemical released by the brain following the digestion of a particular protein called tryptophane. Many of the high protein foods that we eat contain tryptophane but unless we do something to our diet they are digested along with the other proteins we eat and do very little to relieve body ache. When you have attacks of body ache switch your diet to

high carbohydrate and low protein. The carbohydrates will eliminate excess proteins from your body, and leave tryptophane
behind where it will work to activate the endorphins in your brain.
For those who have had chronic body ache a switch to a high
carbohydrate diet has been very effective in getting rid of the
body ache and in replacing it with a feeling of optimism and vigor.

Stay away from alcohol for pain relief. While it can promote the release of endorphins chronic use for this purpose can
result in greater problems. Chocolate works well for many
Americans, although any other sweet food that you like a great
deal might do just as well. If you are a little more physical take
a walk, go for a jog, or take a ride on a bike. Exercise is known
to release endorphins and result in the high many people feel
after a workout. People do get addicted to feeling good, and you
can find a way of achieving this without the use of drugs for most
types of body ache if you will just make use of the natural stim-
ulants of your body's endorphins.

CALCIUM

Calcium is needed for strong bones and teeth. That is
what we are told all of our lives, and it's true. But now new uses
for calcium are being discovered that are very exciting. Calcium
has been found to be effective in preventing cancer, and those
with the highest levels of calcium in their diets also had the low-
est rate of high blood pressure. There is debate as to whether
calcium helps overcome insomnia, so if a warm glass of milk
helps you get to sleep use it, and if it doesn't then try something
else. On the downside calcium can sometimes form kidney
stones causing a great deal of pain and occasionally destroying
a kidney. One of our concerns in looking at calcium supplements
will be to find those that minimize the risk of kidney stones. But
in looking at calcium supplements, the only reason that we have
to be concerned with them is that some people are unable to use
the calcium occurring in dairy products, having a problem called
lactose intolerance. Calcium supplements may also be necessary in cases of certain medical conditions such as pregnancy,

or when there is an inability to absorb calcium from foods. Calcium is necessary all of our lives and it is important to our health to have a dependable source, as well as to know when we need extra calcium and where to get it.

WHAT SUPPLEMENTS CAN DO IF YOU FOLLOW ADVICE

You need to take calcium supplements, of the proper kind, whenever your need for calcium is greater than what your diet supplies. The symptoms of calcium depletion are muscle cramps, problems with your teeth and gums, backaches, aching bones, and any signs of disease which affects the bones, hair, or teeth. The proper calcium supplements can prevent all of these problems as well as help prevent osteoporosis, and speed up the process of healing in broken bones. Pregnant women should always take calcium supplements both to ensure the health of their baby as well as to prevent the growth of the baby from stealing calcium from their bodies. If you are taking steroid drugs, or you drink alcohol, calcium supplements should be included to prevent depletion. Adequate calcium will ensure good hair and fingernails, as well as healthy bones and teeth. Since we have no storage reservoirs of calcium, except for our hair, bones and teeth, those areas with the greatest need are going to steal calcium from those with a lesser need. That is why a baby may be born with good calcium levels at the same time that the mother is developing calcium deficiency. Extra calcium, in most forms in which we get it, is simply flushed out of our body through our kidneys. However, we can't take just any supplement and expect it to help us over a special need or to prevent a chronic problem. If we choose the wrong supplement they may not do any good at all, and that happens more often than we like to believe.

WHY SUPPLEMENTS OFTEN DON'T DO ANY GOOD

A common reason why supplements are ineffective is that they are just inadequate. After all, how do you know how much calcium to take, even if you know you should take it? Since some supplements are toxic at high levels, you may be afraid to take enough calcium to help you with your particular problem. A little guide may be helpful: 600 mg if you are healthy, get plenty of exercise, and are not pregnant or in the process of healing from a broken bone; 1200 mg if you have a less than perfect diet, don't exercise regularly, have occasional muscle cramping, are pregnant or nursing, or have older relatives who have suffered from osteoporosis; and 1600 mg if you have osteoporosis, have leg cramps at night, have a broken bone that is healing, or if you are taking steroid drugs.   The supplements are meant to relieve and assist the healing of these problems. Of course if you have osteoporosis calcium supplements are not going to correct the condition, but they are meant to slow and stop the progress of the problem to save further deterioration of your bones. If you take inadequate amounts of calcium when you have these problems there will be no relief and you may think that the supplements are ineffective when it is really the dose that is too low.

Calcium supplements may also be ineffective if they are the wrong type.   Not all calcium supplements are taken by mouth. Some are also taken as shots into the veins or into the muscles. If you are administering your own supplements, and buying them without a doctor's oversight you may be using the wrong type for the method of administration that you are using. As a rule you should never give yourself anything except oral supplements. The oral forms are calcium chloride, calcium gluconate, calcium lactate, and precipitated calcium carbonate. For side effects though the precipitated calcium carbonate can cause constipation, calcium chloride can cause irritation of the digestive tract, and none of these should be used in doses of more than 1600 mg per day.

CALCIUM SUPPLEMENTS WITH LEAD, WHAT TO USE INSTEAD

You are most in danger of having your calcium supplement contaminated with lead if you depend on natural sources.

Since lead collects in the bones, if you use a natural bone meal supplement you may also be getting a dose of lead along with your calcium. If you want to use natural sources read the labels to see if contaminants are listed. Since all natural sources have contaminants there should be some entries. Do not tolerate any lead in the forms you use.

If I found it impossible to find a natural source of calcium supplement without lead I would resort to a chemically based form. While those who prefer natural foods and medicines believe that the trace elements which accompany the main ther- apeutic vitamin or mineral are needed for your body, in the case of lead you do not want to get any dose that you can avoid. The lead tolerance level in the body is zero. Lead collects in the bones and will develop serious disease according to the level it reaches. Because we all live in a world where lead has been used in paints and gasoline in the near past, and even in the pre- sent, every one of us has lead in our bones. We can't get rid of it, but we can avoid getting any more than we have to. Don't use any food or vitamin sources that are likely to have lead.

CANCER

Cancer is a disease in which some of our cells grow out of control. They grow too fast, they don't grow where they should, they simply grow until they stop up vital organs and either kill or disable us. You can never ignore cancer if you get it, and you can get it in many ways. Smoking has always been the major cause of lung cancer as well of several other forms of cancer. Women are subject to breast cancer and cervical can- cer just as a result of living. In fact all cancers become more fre- quent the longer we live. This has led to the conclusion that can- cer is caused by the buildup of cancer causing elements in our bodies. In fact it is thought by some doctors that we are being attacked by cancer cells throughout most of our lives, and when something happens to our immune system so that it doesn't overcome the cancer cells we develop cancer. Once started it is not known if it can be cured again by the body. Cancer requires treatment by a doctor, but fighting the causes of cancer can be done by every one of us every day. Not everyone gets cancer no matter how old the population. Cancer is not the most common disease of old age, and is not the major killer we have to face. Cancer has been successfully resisted by most of us, and with some help maybe the rest of us have a chance to keep from developing cancer in the first place.

FOODS THAT FIGHT OFF CANCER CELLS AND INHIBIT THEIR GROWTH

There are many foods that fight off cancer cells, and many of them are specific to particular kinds of cancer. I will give you a few of the best overall cancer fighters, and then a short selection of each of the others for particular kinds of cancer.

General cancer fighters include whole grains, broccoli, carrots and lettuce.

Bladder cancer fighters are spinach, oranges, cantaloupe, and squash.

Breast cancer fighters are corn, cabbage, whole wheat, beans, peas, and vegetable oils.

Cervical and vaginal cancer fighters are yeast, soy beans, oats, whole wheat, and brown rice.

Colon cancer fighters are vegetables, fruit, and grain.

Lung cancer fighters are dark green vegetables such as spinach, and broccoli.

Skin cancer fighters are carrots, yams, spinach, squash, and cantaloupe.

3 PROVEN CANCER PREVENTING FOODS

Rather than introduce some new cancer preventing foods I would like to tell you about 3 of the foods that you see more than once in the lists above, and why they are such good cancer preventing foods. With a little information you can not

these foods with more understanding, but you can
ditional choices to vary your diet and maximize your
r preventing cancer.

. Broccoli has recently been discovered by cancer prevention nutritionists, after having long been ignored as a vegetable with much interest. The first contribution to cancer prevention by broccoli is beta carotene, of which it delivers 2500 IU
in a 4 once portion. Beta carotene promotes the utilization of vitamin A which fights degenerative diseases including cancer.
Beta carotene, and the foods that supply it provide a barrier
between your body and cancer cells.

2. Whole wheat is good for so many things that it is not
surprising that it is also effective in fighting some types of cancer. Whole wheat contains about 0.13 mg of selenium in a 4
once portion.   Selenium is effective against breast cancer
according to studies noting selenium levels and breast cancer
cases. The higher the level of selenium in the diet the lower the
breast cancer rate. Whole wheat is also an excellent source of
folic acid, which fights the development of cervical and vaginal
cancers, and of vitamin E which fights skin cancer. Whole wheat
should be in everyone's diet to combat cancer, as well as for the
many other benefits it can give.

3. Spinach, the Popeye food, is no longer promoted as a
good source of iron, although its new roll in cancer prevention is
more important anyway.. While you may not think of spinach as
anything more than a type of lettuce, it contains substantial
amounts of vitamin C, folic acid, beta carotene, and vitamin E.
While the levels of these cancer fighters is not as high in spinach
as in certain other cancer fighting foods, it contain so many elements beneficial against cancer that it should be included as a
regular part of every diet.

CATARACTS

A cataract is not a particular disease, since it can have
many causes, but it is a particular condition. Any time the lens
of the eye clouds up so that we can't see clearly out of it we have

developed a cataract. Causes include diseases, radiation, and direct injury to the eye. But the most common forms are characterized by nutritional deficiencies affecting the eyes. In nutrition certain parts of the body have preference over other parts, and for many of our body systems trace elements are responsible for healthy operating, and this includes the eyes. Healthy eyes require adequate amounts of vitamin A, vitamin B-2, calcium, vitamin D, and vitamin E. While cataracts are one of the most serious problems we can have with our eyes, to keep them healthy and resistant against all eye diseases we need to include adequate amounts of each of these nutrients in our diet.

HOW TO CUT RISKS BY AT LEAST 50%

The formation of cataracts is associated with a deficiency of vitamin C. Studies have found that cataracts form 30 times slower when adequate amounts of vitamin C are included in the diet. While vitamin C is found widely in fruits and vegetables, the best sources are oranges, spinach, and green peppers. Artificial sources are also widely available for reasonable prices, but fresh natural sources are not that much more expensive, and all seem to have benefits other than giving you a dose of vitamin C. Other vital nutrients needed to prevent the development of cataracts are vitamin D, vitamin B-2, and Calcium.

The mechanism by which vitamin C resists cataracts is not known, it is only known that there is a direct relationship in the diet and the rate at which cataracts form. Vitamin D and calcium work together in that adequate calcium seems to prevent cataract formation, and vitamin D is necessary for the body to utilize calcium properly. The relationship to vitamin B-2 is known less well. It is just that cataracts are found much more frequently in individuals with a B-2 deficiency, and the logical conclusion is that following a diet high in B-2 may be beneficial in preventing cataract formation.

DIETARY TREATMENTS

If you have read the entry just before this you know what

types of food I am going to recommend: foods high in vitamin C, vitamin D, calcium, and vitamin B-2. Choose from among the list for a daily dose of the essential anti-cataract nutrients, in milligrams per 4 once serving.

Vitamin C: green peppers, 110; strawberries, 52; spinach, 51; oranges, 50, cabbage, 47; grapefruit, 38; cantaloupe, 33; tomatoes, 23; squash, 22; and pineapple, 17.

Vitamin D: sardines, 500; tuna, 250; eggs, 48; cheese, 30; milk and cottage cheese, 4.

Calcium: cheese, 700; sardines, 350; beans, 130; milk, 120; walnuts, 99; and spinach, 93.

Vitamin B-2: liver, 4.1; almonds, 0.92; cheese, 0.46; chicken, 0.36; eggs, 0.28; cottage cheese, 0.25; beans, 0.22; and spinach, broccoli, and beef, 0.20.

These are not all of the foods that supply a significant level of these nutrients. The lists given here are only meant as a guide so that you can be certain of getting them into your diet. If you have a well varied diet which includes meat, dairy products, and several servings of fruit, vegetables, and whole grains every day it is unlikely that you have a dietary deficiency in any of these necessary anti-cataract nutrients.

CERVICAL CANCER

Cervical cancer is one of the number one killers of women in the United States. Unless a woman is checked regularly by a doctor cervical cancer can develop to the point that it will kill her before she even knows she has it. Just the fact that the woman's cervix is inside her body and cannot be examined without effort, it makes it more difficult to see diseases in this area.

Granting that women will never have perfect care of this area of their bodies it is important that they take some precautions to protect themselves from getting cervical cancer in the first place. This may do more to save women from dying from this disease than all of the ads run by the government telling them to get regular checkups. While the ads should still be run, and all women who can should get the checkups as recommended, those women who take steps to protect themselves through diet should be better off on average than women who depend entirely upon the checkups to protect them against cervical cancer.

HOW TO LOWER THE RISK 80% WITH DIET

The best protective nutrient again cervical cancer is folic acid. In a comparative study of women with a condition called dysplasia, which is a precursor to cervical cancer, the women taking folic acid had their dysplasia arrested or reversed. Women taking a placebo had no relief or reversals. The case is pretty solid for folic acid as a preventive of cervical cancer no matter what your history of exposure to cancer causing agents. In further tests, which could not define if the nutrients were actually protective, it was found that women with normal pap smears had higher levels of beta carotene and vitamin C than did women with abnormal pap smears, and cervical dysplasia. The evidence is suggestive that a deficiency of beta carotene and vitamin C may promote the development of cervical cancer.

Folic acid is found widely in our diets, but usually in very small amounts. This is the problem. If we are trying to protect you from a disease where causes are not clearly known, and we don't know when you may be exposed to something that can result in the beginning of a cancer, how well can you be protected if your folic acid intake varies from near zero to a satisfactory level on a day to day basis? So, although you may decide on a folic acid supplement to ensure your intake amount, there are probably many of you who would like to use natural sources as well. With that in mind I will give you the best sources I have for dietary folic acid. The foods listed, are followed by the number of milligrams of folic acid per 4 once serving, and your goal should be 10 milligrams of folic acid per day for maximum protection. Soy beans, 0.69; oats, 0.39; beans, 0.31; liver, 0.31; whole wheat, 0.22; brown rice, 0.17; asparagus, 0.12; and spinach, 0.080.

Now I also mentioned beta carotene and vitamin C, and lists of good sources have been given before so they don't really need to be given again here. No prescribed level has been established for beta carotene, but for vitamin C you should have at least 90 milligrams per day. For specific sources look at the list under cataracts, that was given a few paragraphs before.

CHEAP FOODS VERSES EXPENSIVE PRESCRIPTIONS FOR SAFE TREATMENT OF ILLNESS

Everyone knows that prescriptions are taken to treat illness. The procedure in using a prescription is that you develop an illness, you go and see a doctor, he writes out a prescription to treat the illness, and you go and buy the prescription and take it to cure the illness or relieve the symptoms. At the point where you become dependent upon a prescription to treat your illness you begin paying whatever is demanded by the drug makers, and for many prescription drugs they will charge you $50 to $100 a month for treatment. If your treatment is chronic the cost of prescriptions can literally drive you out of your home. You will be making decisions as to whether you should eat for the month or take the prescriptions.

Compared to the price of most prescriptions food is cheap. What isn't realized most of the time is that food is also the source of many of the medicines that we find in prescriptions. We aren't quite so aware of this in the United States because all of our medicines hide behind Latin names and the names of drug companies. But in China and the rest of Asia the medicines are called by the names of the foods they are taken from. In general, Chinese medicine is just as effective as Western medicine, but the cost is much less.

If we can take a lesson from the Chinese, eating a diet according to their prescriptions for proper nutrition also gives them daily doses of the medicines they are prescribed should they become sick. Now the American diet was once based in the same sort of logic. People would manage their health with fresh foods and home care, and doctors were not treated like gods. The costs of health were very low compared to what they are today, and there was really nothing like the medical industry we have now.

We can get back to this way of managing many of our diseases if we educate ourselves. We have to know what foods to use for which illnesses, and we have to know when to go to the doctor and give ourselves up to prescription medicines. I can't give you a final answer on replacing prescriptions with a good diet, but I can say that if you are careful about what you eat when you are sick you might avoid some of those visits to the doctor, and his ever present prescriptions for medicine that you pay for even if they do more harm than good.

CHEST PAIN RELIEF

We have already looked at some long term relief from angina using hawthorne and chrysanthemum. While these work over time, I can also give you something that should work for chest pain, and it can be found in any supermarket. Get yourself a juicer and start drinking daily glasses of raw fruit and vegetable juices. In one test it took about a month for the effect, but at the end of that time a man with chronic chest pain woke up pain free. He had been using up to 20 nitroglycerine tablets a day, and they were becoming progressively ineffective.

If you want to try this man's raw juice cocktail for chest pain I can give you his prescription: 10 tablespoons of wheat germ oil, 1/2 cup of carrot juice, 1/2 cup of lettuce juice, and one teaspoon of lemon juice. I won't say that this is the only good recipe for a raw juice drink, and you should modify it according to your needs and the effect it has on you. Once you start it give it time.

When you start using raw juices you lose a lot of the fiber that is found naturally in the fruits and vegetables. Now while you may want the fiber for your digestive health, you may need the vitamins and mineral even more. You can still eat raw fruits and vegetables, but you will be supercharging your body with all of the vitamins and minerals that you would ordinarily lose in cooking and storing. Try a raw juice cocktail each day if you suffer from chest pain and with a little luck you may be able to avoid becoming dependent on pills the doctor gives you.

CHOLESTEROL

Cholesterol is a necessary substance in our body. It is found in much of our food, and if we don't eat it our body manufacturers it. The downside of cholesterol is that it is implicated in hardening of the arteries, strokes, and heart attacks. Cholesterol in the blood, when it gets to too high of a level, coats the arteries until it stops the blood from flowing properly. When the arteries block up we end up with a heart attack or stroke.

Luckily not all cholesterol is bad, or bad for you. It has been found that cholesterol comes in two forms, high density cholesterol and low density cholesterol, or HDL and LDL. The HDL form is actually beneficial to us, and just measuring the overall cholesterol level is no longer satisfactory to decide if there is a risk.   The important numbers now are the ratio between the HDL and LDL cholesterol. The higher the proportion of HDL to LDL the better off we are.

Don't ignore your cholesterol levels the next time a doctor gives them to you, but make sure you ask about the ratio of HDL to LDL before you make any decisions as to steps to take in regard to the level.

In warning I also want to tell you that although cholesterol lowering drugs do decrease the level of cholesterol in your blood, they also have side effects that may be worse than the high cholesterol. If you have high cholesterol work on finding a preventive diet to lower the levels to normal. Using the drug company's solutions may kill you. But we will start with a simple step you can take in the form of a cooking spice. Since you probably already have this in your spice rack you could begin using it right now.

TREATMENT WITH A COOKING SPICE

If you like spicy food you're in luck because cayenne pepper is an excellent treatment for lowering cholesterol. Of course cayenne can be added to cold foods as well as hot ones, but most everyone has it in their kitchen cabinet. Cayenne does its work by promoting the excretion of cholesterol. While we don't know exactly how it works, we do know that cayenne, along with other hot peppers, also works as a pain reliever, helps blood clotting, and relieves the discomfort of arthritis. The work that cayenne does on cholesterol may not be as obvious, but over the long run it may be more important than the help it can give in solving the more obvious problems.

FOODS THAT HELP LOWER YOUR CHOLESTEROL

I have already mentioned that cayenne pepper can lower cholesterol, but there are many other foods that work just as well. I want you to have a selection to make it possible to include some of them in your diet every day. With this in mind I will give you a dozen foods that lower cholesterol through several different mechanisms. Using natural foods to lower cholesterol is always better than depending upon medications for the same purpose since foods do not have the side effects of pharmaceutical medications. To get an idea of how effective your diet is in lowering cholesterol just choose those foods listed before and add the percent instead of subtracting them to see what your cholesterol level would be if you had no good eating habits. If you have a good diet today, changing it to a more typical American diet could result in a rise in cholesterol by 50% or more.

An apple a day keeps the doctor away. Whether that is true or not 2 or 3 apples a day can reduce cholesterol by 10%. It is best to space your apple eating throughout the day. The benefit of apples to lower cholesterol is more than just lowering your overall cholesterol, it also results in a rise in LDL cholesterol, and a drop in HDL cholesterol. Many doctors believe that the relative amounts of these two types of cholesterol is even more important than your overall cholesterol level in maintaining a healthy heart.

Everyone loves Mexican food, but does it do anything for cholesterol? Actually it does, and it is the beans that make up so much of the Mexican food diet that is most effective in lowering cholesterol. Research has found that as little as one cup of beans a day will lower cholesterol by 19%. Of course Mexican dishes use pinto beans, but the effect has also been found in baked and canned beans as well. The wonderful effect of beans on cholesterol are believed to be the result of the fiber they contain. Other than high fiber, beans tend to be high in proteins, and vary in vitamins and minerals. Beans also cause a favorable shift in the LDL and HDL cholesterol ratios.

Carrots are good for the eyes, but they are also good in lowering cholesterol. If you eat 3 medium carrots a day you are lowering your cholesterol by about 11%.

Milk should not be cut out of your diet if you have high cholesterol, just switch to skim milk. Several studies have noted a drop in cholesterol levels when diets include daily use of skim milk. Although no arguments have been put forth to explain this drop in cholesterol, I believe it occurs because milk has many important nutrients, and when you use skim milk you aren't adding cholesterol to your body while you are getting your basic nutrition.

Oat bran was the champion of the fiber foods just a few years ago. But like many fads it has gone out of fashion so far as write-ups in the tabloids. Nevertheless it is a wonderful source of fiber. Oat bran is water soluble, making it easy to add to many foods, and having a daily dose can lower cholesterol by 19%.

We all need to use oils in cooking now and then, or over a salad, and that is as good a reason as any to keep olive oil in your kitchen. Olive oil and cholesterol have been studied at the Center for Human Nutrition at the University of Texas in Dallas, and it was found that a daily use of at least 2 teaspoons will keep cholesterol within normal levels.

Onions are avoided by many people because they do not

like the odor on their breath, or they have trouble digesting them. Personally I like onions very much. They are excellent for fiber, as are most fruits and vegetables, and they lower cholesterol levels, and improve the ratio of HDL to LDL cholesterol.

Seafood of all kinds is promoted as a source of phosphorous and low fat protein. The use in cholesterol is not that it lowers the levels, but that it prevents them from seesawing up and down according to the meals that you have. For best effect seafoods should be eaten several times a week.

Soybeans are the basis of soy sauce, and that is all that many people know about it. Of course you may just not be aware that you can also get soy milk, lecithin, and tofu, which are made from soybeans, and soybeans are the basis of non-meat burgers and sausages that are being sold in the markets at this time. The value in soybean products is that they can help those who have high cholesterol levels now. By high levels I mean 300 or more, which is considered a potentially deadly level by doctors. A diet that consistently contains soy products will cause a drop of 15% to 20% in cholesterol levels.

Spinach, which keeps popping up in this book, though not for iron, is nevertheless an effective cholesterol fighter. Spinach has not been studied in this country, but Japanese studies using animals found cholesterol reduced on a spinach diet.

Yams are not just a holiday food. Personally I like to make a meal of yams every once in a while, and they can always be used to add some natural sweetness to your diet. However, yams are loaded with a very beneficial form of fiber which binds with cholesterol in the diet so that it can pass through the body instead of entering the blood stream. Maybe there is a reason for having yams along with large, cholesterol laden, holiday meals.

Yogurt is a good choice for dietary foods that lower cholesterol since it is a good way to finish off a meal. Yogurt can also make a meal or a snack at any time, and you will know that you are helping your cholesterol level at the same time. Regular use of yogurt has been found to lower cholesterol by 5% to 10% a week, as well as improve the ratio of HDL to LDL cholesterol.

If you like yogurt what better reason do you have to indulge yourself regularly.

NO CHOLESTEROL FOODS THAT ARE ACTUALLY BAD FOR YOU

While the levels of cholesterol in the blood is related pretty closely to the fat we eat, not all fat has the same effect on our cholesterol levels. Saturated fats result in high HDL levels which leads to atheroschlerosis, heart attacks, and strokes. On the other other hand foods that contain non saturated fats may be considered cholesterol free, and yet have a great number of calories from unsaturated fats. With the growth of vegetable oils in cooking, such foods as french fries and fried vegetables are now cholesterol free. But that does not mean they are necessarily good for us?

I don't think so since calories also translate into weight gain, and weight all by itself can contribute to heart attacks and diabetes. Fish, not being a red meat, is also free of cholesterol. But some fish is very high in fat, and also contributes to all of the problems of weight gain.

Fat is not the only problem though, what about sugar. Some candy and other foods may be almost entirely sugar, and cholesterol free, and have a very bad effect on your teeth. Sugar has also been studied in relation to being a cause of cancer although no direct links have been found.

Cholesterol is not the only villain that we have to look out for, as can be seen in the case of sugar and unsaturated fat that is noted here. In addition many Americans depend upon white bread as a basic part of their diets. After all bread is good for you so shouldn't white bread be just as good as any other kind? The answer is no. While white bread may be made with added fiber and vitamins and minerals, it doesn't make up for the fact that the flour in white bread is harder to digest than the flour made from whole grains. This difference can have an effect on your digestive system in such a way that you may develop constipation.

The point I am trying to make is that cholesterol is not the only thing that we have to be concerned about. We have several systems in our body besides our system of blood transport, and we can get just as sick from abusing them as we can if we have a high cholesterol diet all of our lives. While we must certainly be concerned about cholesterol, don't let it be your only concern. Have a well mixed diet, low in cholesterol and red meat, and high in a variety of fruits and vegetables.

CLOGGED ARTERIES

Clogged arteries are otherwise known as atheroschlerosis, and the substance clogging those arteries is cholesterol. Cholesterol clogs arteries by sticking to them as it circulates in the blood. Doctors believe that there are things in the blood that make the cholesterol sticky, and that if they can be controlled then even if you have a high cholesterol diet it will not stick to your arteries and close them up. There is some evidence from people who are known to have high cholesterol levels in the blood, but who rarely suffer strokes or heart attacks. Doctors are even developing a pill that anyone can take that will protect them from their high cholesterol diets.

But that is in the future. Right now you are going to have to do something yourself to take care of the arteries that you have clogged. Of course the doctors have solutions. The most radical is to operate on you, open the clogged arteries, and remove the clogging material directly. Other solutions from the medical community include heart bypass operations, or just giving you blood thinning medications to keep the blood from clotting. If your artery is only clogged in a very limited area doctors sometimes operate and insert a little balloon which pushes the clog open to let the blood flow through normally. All of these solutions, that we get from our wonderful medical community, have risks of complications and death. Once you start taking medications to keep clogged arteries open many doctors will want you to stay on it for the rest of your life.

If you aren't satisfied with this set of options there is one other that you might consider. Diet is often one of the original causes of clogged arteries, and diet can be used to help open them up. There is no guarantee that diet will cure a severe case of clogged arteries, but there are no guarantees with any of the other procedures either. What diet can do is put you back in charge of your health, and it can give you a chance to treat a very serious medical condition that has to be treated in some manner if you are to survive. In order to help you make some decisions on your health I will present a few foods that can help to open the arteries. It will be up to you to choose what you want to try, and to decide if they work for you.

FOODS THAT CAN OPEN THE ARTERIES

In the section on the arteries closing up I have already talked about the use of whole grains in opening up the arteries, and preventing clogging. In this section I would like to give you the foods with the best vitamins for opening the arteries. Of course the two views should be put together for a complete picture of how to manage your arteries, but giving each as a separate approach gives you choices, and you can try one or the other or both.

The best vitamins for healthy arteries are vitamin C, vitamin E, and vitamin B-6. These vitamins are effective because they prevent the blood from clotting in arteries that have been clogged by cholesterol deposits. Now, the best foods to use to get these vitamins to as high a level as possible are the foods that can open the arteries and keep them flowing safely.

Vitamin C can be most abundantly derived from eating acerola cherries. but should your access to these cherries be limited other excellent sources of vitamin C include guavas, green peppers, strawberries, spinach, oranges, cabbage, grapefruit, cantaloupe, green onions, tomatoes, squash, and romaine lettuce.

Vitamin E is best taken in wheat germ if you can get a few ounces of it into your diet every day. Alternative sources, which are also very useful, include sunflower seeds, whole wheat, walnuts, corn oil, hazel nuts, soy and peanut oil, almonds, olive oil, cabbage, peanuts, cashews, spinach, asparagus, broccoli, oats, barley, and corn.

Vitamin B-6, one of the famous B vitamins, does not have an outstanding source. But it does have several fairly good source which are all useful. Beginning with brewer's yeast, and on to brown rice, whole wheat, soybeans, lentils, sunflower seeds, hazelnuts, salmon, wheat germ, tuna, bran, walnuts, peas, liver, avocados, beans, cashews, peanuts, turkey, oats, chicken, been, and bananas.

I trust that I have given you enough choices for these most valuable foods to keep the arteries open. As you can see some of the them have all three vitamins in decent levels, and some appear only once. I do not believe that anyone can eat the same thing at every meal, and I do not advise you to try it. Pick and choose from these lists to include some of the foods each day from each list and you should be able to make thousands of meals without repeating any pattern for years.

COLDS AND FLU

Colds and the flu are mostly seasonal illnesses that bother us in the cold weather months. Summer colds are something else different altogether, and are more likely allergies than diseases. But it is difficult to avoid catching colds a couple of times a year, and the flu nearly every year, when you live in any kind of a city.

While the only sure way to keep from catching these diseases is to stay away from people, there are plenty of ways to relieve the symptoms once you do catch them. Over the counter medicine offers some relief, but there is no reason that you can't just use foods to accomplish the same thing. My philosophy about food and medicine is that if you can find a diet that will control a medical problem then use that instead of going to the drug store and looking for the same thing in a package. It is very rare for anyone to have side effects from treatments they have gotten through their diets, while medications from the pharmaceutical companies always carry the possibility of problems from side effects. In relation to colds and the flu it may take a little creativity to find the right foods for relief, but the effort is well worth while.

DRINKS AND FOODS TO SPEED RELIEF

For many years Linus Pauling, the Noble prize winner, researched and promoted the use of vitamin C to relieve and prevent colds and the flu. While the AMA never widely accepted Pauling's statements on the effectiveness of vitamin C against colds and the flu, his evidence is very strong that a daily dose of 70 milligrams or more of vitamin C will lower the number of colds and your chance of getting the flu by 30% to 40%. Pauling also found that high doses of vitamin C can shorten the time you have a cold or the flu, and seemed to relieve the symptoms as well. While you can't get doses in the thousands from natural foods very easily, it is possible to get a few hundred milligrams a day if you choose a high vitamin C diet. So for cold and flu prevention with vitamin C include some of the foods listed below every day. After each food is a number giving the milligrams of vitamin C you will get in a 4 once serving. Vitamin C: green peppers, 110; strawberries, 52; spinach, 51; oranges, 50, cabbage, 47; grapefruit, 38; cantaloupe, 33; tomatoes, 23; squash, 22; and pineapple, 17.

But to get away from the vitamin people for a bit, people have used a lot of common foods to fight colds for many years, and just in case you don't include them in your diet now I will tell you a little about them.

I will start with one that everyone has heard of but most people seem to forget about when they get sick. Chicken soup, a standard Jewish joke, actually works quite well to relieve stuffiness and end the symptoms of a cold. Of course any other soup may do just as well, but the Jewish community has depended on it for so many years that maybe there is something special about chicken soup. Personally I would rather have a warm bowl of chicken soup if I had a bad cold or the flu than one of those 12-hour cold tablets.

Onions and garlic both have been used for cold remedies, and since these are also proposed as anti-cancer foods and digestion aids, it is possible that they are effective with colds and the flu as well. To use an onion, or garlic, it should be well cooked, that is very well cooked. It can be ingested with a soup or straight if you wish. The dose is one medium onion or two cloves of garlic a day. Cooking onions and garlic well before eating them makes them easier to digest, and should help those who have never had much of either of these excellent vegetables in their diets.

Besides the congestion fighters just mentioned you should also use zinc, and vitamin A, vitamin E, and vitamin B complex. Without giving you a rundown of each specific food to eat for high doses of each of these I can still give you some advice that will add up to a high intake of all of them. First, you need a varied diet which should be rich in vegetables and whole grains. When you are sick with a cold or the flu you may lose your appetite. Even if you do, you need to eat whole grain cereals, preferably hot, along with home made vegetable soups, and cooked vegetables. Stay away from oil cooked foods and raw vegetables at this time since they will add calories and difficulty in digestion. A nice, well done, vegetable stew is a good choice. Meats should be eaten sparingly, and avoid fatty foods.

COLON CANCER

Colon cancer should be considered a silent killer since most of the time you don't know about it until it has spread to other parts of the body. Colon cancer occurs in the digestive system, and diet is largely believed to contribute to its formation. Diets that seem to cause colon cancer are high in fats, refined sugars and flour, and low in fiber, whole grains, and fresh fruits and vegetables. While someone who eats one type of foods may also eat the other, the more to one side or the other that you are the greater or the lesser is your risk of getting colon cancer.

The medical establishment recommends a regular checkup of your digestive tract to protect you from colon cancer. But they also recommend increasing vegetables and fruit, and decreasing fat and sugar. To this we very much agree, except that since it is very likely that diet is at the root cause of colon cancer, it can also be at the root of its prevention. While you can lower your risk of colon cancer with a diet that is high in the right kinds of foods and low in those that increase risk, you can also decrease your risk by 30% just by ensuring that you have an adequate intake of a dietary mineral, and that is what I would like to talk about at this time.

LOWER YOUR RISK WITH A DIETARY MINERAL

You may have heard how yogurt helps to prevent colon cancer by keeping the digestive bacteria healthy. Well there may be another aspect to the effectiveness of yogurt that could explain a few other things as well. Along with digestive bacteria yogurt also has a good dose of calcium, and it has been found that calcium, when combined with vitamin D, is also associated with low colon cancer rates. Looking through the books and reports on colon cancer prevention it always seems a little odd that acidophalus milk should be so effective against colon cancer. Now it may be that the acidophalus itself is a cancer fighter, or that the bacteria it removed is a cause of cancer, which is possible, but I think that the real effectiveness lies in the high calcium content of milk. Perhaps those who use acidophalus milk also use low fat or no fat varieties, which also cuts down on a major cancer causing agent.

Preliminary studies have found that a high calcium diet does carry a 30% lower risk of developing colon cancer, when combined with a high level of vitamin D. It has even been speculated that the lower rate of colon cancer experienced by New Yorkers who move to Florida is the result of increased vitamin D from being outside more than the New Yorkers they leave behind. This does make sense, and I certainly see nothing harmful in having low fat, or non-fat, milk products in your diet, and you getting some exercise in the sun on a regular basis. The exercise alone should do you good since exercise has been found to decrease cancer rates as well.

CONSTIPATION

Is constipation the illness nobody wants to talk about? It may very well be. How long has it been since your casual conversations with your friend has turned to how often they have suffered from constipation. While constipation is not a polite disease, it is a common disease. I have a friend whose family suffers from, what I consider to be, a lot of constipation. I have been told on more than one occasion that some member of his family has had constipation. I strongly suspect that for every such episode that he has related to me there are probably 4 or 5 more. I may be wrong, but the number of times he has talked to me about this is 100% higher than the number of times I have found the problem in my own household.

Constipation has also reared its ugly head in relation to this persons career. In each of the last several years he has experienced violent digestive problems as he has returned to his career after his summer vacation. While they have not been largely serious, they have caused him a lot of pain, and I always fear that there may be a serious illness one day.

While my friend may react to the stress of returning to his job badly, there is no reason that it should be expressed as a digestive problem unless there is something wrong with his diet to begin with. Since his problems are shared by his family on a somewhat frequent basis I believe that the overall cause lies in the family diet.

I have dined with him and his family from time to time and I have found their diet to contain a high level of fat and refined sugar and flour, some fresh fruits, and no raw or cooked vegetables. At least none worth mentioning. I do not see any way out of concluding that the periodic problems of constipation experienced by this family are not related to their diet. If you do not get sufficient roughage in your diet, and you get an abundance of fat and refined foods, your digestive system will not process the food you eat at a normal rate. By decreasing one you increase the other. In other words, if you have constipation you have probably caused it through your diet.

But, even supposing you have taken some precautions

against getting constipation by decreasing your fats you have still gotten constipation, what can you do?   There are many courses you can take short of resorting to the use of medications that promote bowel movements or other such medications. You can still act on your own, and without cost, if you follow the suggestions that are given here in regard to a natural drink that may be able to end the problem.

A NATURAL DRINK THAT ENDS THE PROBLEM

What is necessary for good digestion. Fiber, bulk, anything else? Actually there is something else. For good digestion you also need to have enough water to keep everything moving through your digestive system. Our bodies are about 90% water anyway, and wherever you have water as part of the bodily function it makes up closer to 98% or 99%. With this in mind it is often a lack of water in the digestive system that results in constipation.

This should not be too surprising since many people do not drink water, or other liquids regularly through the day as they might have done a few years ago. Water is often not even considered a drink to have when you are thirsty, and when you drink sugared drinks at these times the sugars in the drinks make them less able to satisfy your thirst. When you are thirsty you should have water.

Probably the most common single problem with the digestive system is just the amount of water we drink. If you have your 8 glasses of water a day you should avoid most problems of constipation no matter what your diet. Think about it this way. If you have a diet of refined flour you have lost most of its ability to carry water. It is a very dry product, look into your flour sack and see how dry it looks, and to digest it you need enough water in your digestive tract to keep it in a dissolved and liquid state. If your intestinal tract gets dried out by the foods you eat the food will form clumps and you will have constipation.

Advice to avoid constipation, for everyone no matter what the diet, drink water with each meal and between meals. While I don't think that 8 glasses of water is needed for each person, since most people probably have only a couple of glasses of water a day, if you try to have 8 you will at least have enough to prevent constipation and keep your digestion in good order.

WHY YOU SHOULD THROW AWAY YOUR OLD CON-STIPATION MEDICINE

Constipation medicines are called cathartics in the medical field. They vary in what they are supposed to do, some irritate the digestive system to get it to work, some just add bulk, and some make things slide more easily. These are the three main methods by which all problems of constipation operate, but with constipation medicines they operate in a concentrated form. The most common source for these medications is the vegetables and fruits that we are told to eat when we are constipated anyway, but without a lot of the substances that have undefined functions.

All this is well and good so far as it goes. The problem is that it doesn't go so far as to seeing why some constipation medicines work for some people and why they don't work for other people. As it turns out because you may use the wrong type of medication for your constipation you may actually make things worse instead of making them better. If you have an irritated colon, and you use an irritant medicine you will not cure anything. The problem is that since you can't see into the area where the constipation is taking place you are never really sure which of the three types of cathartics are best for your condition.

Throw away your constipation medications and use a combination of natural foods, water, and bran to fight your constipation. This costs you nothing and will take effect at least as effectively as any of the medications you can buy. The advantage of these high fiber foods is that they can deliver all three types of constipation relief at the same time, and in large amounts. If one peach doesn't take care of the problem then eat two. I can almost guarantee that no case of constipation will persist for more than a few hours when faced with a variety of fresh fruits and vegetables. Along with the foods drink large amounts of water, and forget the medication.

DENTURE PAIN

Experienced denture wearers do not, as a rule, have denture pain. Therefore those I wish to address are new to the business of wearing dentures, and you are probably having a pretty rough time with it right now. For one thing wearing dentures is in the same league as getting used to depending on any artificial device for some of your bodily functions. They are not going to work as well as your natural teeth no matter how long you wear them, but they can be very serviceable for eating and talking.

The process of getting dentures includes the removal or loss of all of the teeth in the affected area, as you know of course if you are wearing them. With that removal the condition of the gums will change, and any conditioning they have to the pressures of eating and chewing will be lost for a time. Therefore, when you first start to wear dentures they are going to be uncomfortable. That is true for everyone, and you can use basic gum pain methods to relieve the pain at this time.

You can either use some of the over the counter medications sold in local drug stores, or you can try a few food based remedies and handle it from your kitchen. I would say start with drug store medicines, and switch to a food based type when you find one. A West Indian remedy for toothaches, that should work for sore gums as well, is to take the juice of a fresh lime and soak it into a cotton wad. Put the cotton directly on the sore area and within 5 minutes, or even less, the pain should subside. This is completely safe, and limes are only about a dime each. Another simple gum pain reliever can be made from crushed tulip bulbs. Just take a fresh tulip bulb, crush it sufficiently so that it is mashed, and use the mash as a poultice. This brings relief very quickly.

There is one other suggestion I would like to make as to quick and safe pain relief. Take a warm glass of water and dissolve a teaspoon of salt into it. Then gargle with the salt water two or three times, and repeat as necessary to relieve pain. This method can be used for any local pain or sores in the mouth.

Otherwise I would suggest that you just wait and adjust. It will take some time before dentures will be comfortable, and for some people they never stop giving pain. But for most of you, if you use local pain relievers and wait eventually the dentures will be at least tolerable and perform their function without any particular concern on your part.

DEPRESSION

While depression often accompanies personal disasters and burdens, it may not be these problems that cause the depression. There is a field of thought among nutritionists that see nutrition as a sign of borderline malnutrition in certain areas. This doesn't seem quite so unreasonable when you think about it. At times of stress we normally change our eating habits. Some people eat a great deal more than normal, but of foods out of their normal diet, and other people stop eating altogether. These dietary changes add up to a deficiency in many people, but because it may only go on for a few weeks or months it may not be diagnosed before the eating habits have changed again.

Now, be this as it may, this means that many cases of depression can be treated with diet, and that is what we will explore a little bit after we look at the brain chemistry of depression in more detail.

HOW IT IS CAUSED BY BRAIN CHEMISTRY

For a hint as to exactly which vitamins are responsible for depression we can take a look at the menstrual cycle of women. Many women experience a cycle of depression along with their menstrual cycle. But since it does not occur to all women every month we can be certain that it is not part of the menstruation itself, but of something else that women do sometimes and sometimes not. Research has found that the changes in diet, along with menstrual bleeding, leave some women with a borderline deficiency of B vitamins. One of these, vitamin B-6, is especially active in brain chemistry since it interacts with chemicals that control the relay of signals through the brain. Also, those women with the largest drop in vitamin B-6 suffer the most consistent cases of depression. While other studies may be needed to confirm all of this, there is enough evidence here for you to take some action in order to decrease or eliminate depression from this cause.

NATURAL AMINO ACIDS AND DOPAMINE FOR DRUG FREE RELIEF

The amino acids that relieve depression are L-phenylalinine and tyrosine, and doses of 500 to 1000 mg a day for 2 weeks is usually sufficient . High doses of phenylalinine have side effects, and can cause high blood pressure possibly bringing on a stroke or heart attack. Phenylalinine is one of the 8 essential amino acids that we have to get through our diets. Tyrosine is made from phenylalinine by the body, or it can be derived directly from food. To relieve depression naturally with phenylalinine and tyrosine you need to plan a diet high in complete proteins. The best protein foods are egg whites, meat, whole wheat, beans, cottage cheese, and milk. All are complete proteins, and by including one or more of these in each of your meals when you are depressed you should be able to give yourself a phenylalinine boost sufficient to promote the proper brain chemistry to relieve the depression.   Dopamine is then made from tyrosine, and is also necessary for proper brain function. Healthy levels of dopamine promote a normal sleep cycle. In cases of depression one of the most common problem is an inability to sleep normally.

If you experience severe depression put yourself on a high protein diet. You can include meat, or have it meat free, but stress protein at this time over fruit and vegetables. If you are taking care of someone who has experienced a tragedy or other life event that has placed them into a state of depression do everything in your power to get them to eat protein daily. Natural proteins are safer than their chemical derivatives. There is virtually no way for you to overdose on an amino acid with natural proteins. All in all give the diet about 2 weeks before expecting to see results. Of course it may take longer, but 2 weeks is the minimum time doctors follow amino acid therapy with depression before they expect a change in the patients psychological state.

DE-TOXIFYING FOODS

Foods can be toxic either from what is in them, or from what is on them. Some pesticides can enter into a food and make it difficult or impossible to remove. Toxins that are just on the outside of a food can usually be removed by peeling or washing. With modern agriculture it is probably a good idea to consider that the outside of all fresh foods has been sprayed with pesticides, and should be either peeled or washed.

One problem with toxins on food is that you may believe that a food is toxin free when it is really contaminated with pesticides or fertilizer. Now days it is even worse since genetically engineered foods are appearing where the contaminant has become part of the food itself. The only way to avoid these toxic substances is to find a producer who does not use the genetic form. This you may have to do through a health food store since the government is not letting producers advertise that their foods are free of these substances in their supermarket ads. I say that you should take whatever steps are necessary to ensure that you have as few toxins in your diet as possible.

DIABETES

Diabetes, the inability to maintain a proper sugar level in the blood, is thought to be caused largely by diet. At least many cases of diabetes occur where the diet is bad, and overloaded with sugar, alcohol, and refined carbohydrates. Disease and medications are also common causes, but most cases have no known cause, and the only logical conclusion is that something in what we eat or do is the basic cause of the illness.

The typical history of a diabetes sufferer begins in childhood with a diet laced with candy and sweets. The basic family food used refined white flour, and relatively few vegetables and fruits. While the carbohydrates are worthwhile, they usually come with a high level of fat in the form of bakery goods.

As a teenager this person has the normal medical problems, and is heavily indulged in junk foods as they acquire some money of their own. Over the course of the years more meals are had as fast food and fewer as meals produced at home in any form. The nutrition shifts even more towards fat, sugar, and refined flour. This process goes on for 8 or 10 years, and in this period we begin to see a rise in the number of diabetes cases around the country.

In early adulthood diets generally get better. As the search for a spouse, jobs, and the bearing of children is uppermost in these years the concern for health is also at a peak. People take better care of themselves at this time then at any other time of their lives. Bad habits, like drug use, is often abandoned, and fresh fruits and vegetables, along with exercise, may even make its first appearance since the early years of high school. Most people feel very virtuous at some periods of this time, and not unexpectedly new cases of diabetes decline.

In the late 40s and 50s many people reach the height of their affluence. They can indulge in alcohol, rich foods, fancy meats, and meals on the town. With many other concerns out of the way diets and exercise both decline, and general health declines along with it. Diabetes begins to rise and continues to rise through the rest of life. However, diabetes at this time is not the same as what is experienced in the young years. While it has something to do with how the body works, and the hormones and body systems operating, many of these cases do not even require insulin. Dietary management is possible, and self management is often successful.

This broad outline of the course of diabetes through the life of the American population just illustrates the risk we face and how it is related to our diets. By following a good diet throughout our lives, and doing all other things in moderation, we can minimize the risk. You can clean up your act at any time, but the sooner the better. Now I can give you a few ideas that may help even if you currently have some of the bad habits associated with the development of diabetes. One of the major causes is thought to be metal that builds up in your body over time, and there are some foods you should consider that might help to remove them and lower your risk level.

FOODS TO REMOVE METALS FROM YOUR BODY THAT MAY CAUSE DIABETES

Metal play a small but critical role in the complications of diabetes. Metal ions circulate in the blood and play a role in destroying nerve endings and creating other complications. By removing the metal ions you can slow the progress of the disease and prevent many of the problems that you may face.

Since you can't remove all of these metals from your diet, as they are just trace elements anyway, you can add foods that will do the job for you. These foods work by a process called chelation. Chelation binds the metal ions to other molecules than can be more easily removed from the blood. Doctors perform chelation therapy in the hospital using a drip system that puts the concentrated chemicals into your blood, and you may be able to do much the same thing naturally through diet.

If you have a case of uncontrolled diabetes you may not have a choice, but if you have controlled or borderline diabetes you may be able to help control complications by your use of chelation type foods. The effect won't be as intense as you will get from the medical treatment, but the administration can go on for a long period of time, and there are no side effects.

Chelating foods and vitamins are vitamin C, vitamin E, garlic, legumes, and some amino acids. In fact if you design a diet for yourself that is high in these nutrients before you develop diabetes you may be able to protect yourself from developing it in the first place. These nutrient containing foods have been recommended for other purposes in this book, and as you can see here they may prevent another of the diseases of aging, as diabetes is sometimes called. So many of the diseases to which we are subject are associated with poor nutrition the only prudent course is to find a daily diet for yourself that includes several of these foods with each meal. This should provide protection for you over the entire course of your life.

DIARRHEA

Diarrhea goes by many colorful names, but all mean pain and discomfort. Most of the time that we get diarrhea we are doing something unusual, such as going to a picnic, traveling in a foreign country, or taking a new medication. All of this new-ness ads up to exposing our digestive system to foods and bacteria that it is not used to. Of course I can't stop you from get-ting diarrhea with any of my suggestions but maybe I can stop you from getting it so often, and maybe I can help you under-stand enough of the process of getting diarrhea that you can help others to avoid the problem as well.

DIGESTIVE PROBLEMS

Diarrhea is so common it must be unusual if anyone in the country goes a full year without at least one attack of diar-rhea. A minor case of diarrhea may last only a day or less, while a major attack can go on for weeks or months. Luckily for all of us the minor cases are much the majority. This is quite under-standable if we consider the causes.

Most diarrhea is caused by food poisoning, with lesser amounts attributed to reactions to medication, stress, food aller-gies, digestive deficiencies, and various others such as drinking the water in some countries. But since our main concern is diar-rhea in the U.S. we won't worry too much about anything past the first 5 causes.

Food poisoning causes most diarrhea because we can get it every time that we eat, and it comes on within minutes or a few hours of eating something that is contaminated. This also explains why most of these cases are so short. If we have a meal and get sick an hour later we don't go back and eat the same thing again. Chances are we stop eating much of anything for a day or two, and we avoid the probable offending food for months. Thus most food poisoning does not last very long.

Medication is also a common cause of diarrhea because

medicines do things to our bodies other than what we take them for. These are called side effects, and they are usually unpleasant. If we have an infection and take a strong antibiotic to clear it up we are also affecting the bacteria that we have in our digestive system. If you wonder why congestive diseases are so often accompanied by diarrhea it might just be medicine you are treating it with rather than the disease you are treating. With the digestive bacteria destroyed, food does not digest properly, and we often get constipation or diarrhea, and diarrhea seems the most common outcome. These cases of diarrhea last about as long as we are taking strong medications, and often for a day or two longer. The usual recommendation to eat yogurt into order to re-establish the digestive system is a good one. This, along with bulk foods such as bread, rice, and potatoes usually does the job.

Diarrhea from stress is usually very short lived, and is probably also caused by poor eating habits at this time than directly by the stress. Stress causes us to adopt unusual diets, and this often results in diarrhea in many situations. My advice in cases of diarrhea from stress is to take some walks, and plan out a normal and healthy diet. This form of diarrhea should not last for more than a day or two if you maintain a normal diet pattern.

Food allergies work very much like food poisoning. If we eat a food we are allergic to we can develop diarrhea in a matter of an hour, and it will last just so long as we have the food in our system. If the allergy is really severe it can be life threatening. Most food allergies are so mild that they just cause a few symptoms and we avoid the foods that cause them after a little experience. Of course food allergies can crop up at any time, and the most likely time for a new one to find us is when we are trying new foods. Thus, we get diarrhea more often when we are eating foods we are not used to because we may be eating foods we are allergic to. We can't avoid this at all times, but we can minimize it by taking a gulp or two of the pink diarrhea cure we get in the drugstore before having exotic meals. It shouldn't interfere with our enjoyment of the meal, and it can give us some protection against mild food allergies that would result in diarrhea.

Digestive deficiencies include the inability to digest such foods as milk, called lactose deficiency, or other constituents of different foods. Common digestive deficiencies include eggs and chocolate, and you can usually avoid these in their pure form. It is in the mixed foods that we often run into these substances that we can't digest. Eggs show up in most baked goods, but can also appear in many other foods. Chocolate has a difficulty sneaking up on us because it is usually the dominant flavor in any food where it is used. The problem with chocolate is our friends. Most people love chocolate so much that they will encourage their non-digestive friends to have a bit of the chocolate dessert, and they often do and they pay for it. Milk is the same in character as eggs, it is just found everywhere and we often don't know when we are getting it. Inability to digest milk is common around the world, and it is only in such countries as the United States, where we have a huge milk industry, that we think everyone should drink milk all of their lives. The truth is we don't have to drink milk past our first few years. If you like milk anyway, but can't tolerate it, find a good soy milk substitute. The taste may be a little different than cow's milk, but there will be no diarrhea. Soy milk was developed to take care of those milk lovers who could no longer drink cow's milk.

3 FRUITS TO BANISH DIGESTIVE PROBLEMS

There are many foods that are effective in combating digestive problems, including diarrhea, but not many of these are fruits. Fruit, because of its high fiber content, is usually thought to speed digestion rather than slow it and put it in order. For this reason most people avoid all fruit when they are suffering from diarrhea, but this is a mistake. The medicines used in diarrhea medicines are often taken from common dietary fruits and vegetables. All that you need is a guide to some of these original sources and you can go a long way towards treating yourself.

An excellent fruit to control diarrhea is bananas. Bananas are a starchy fruit to begin with, which is a little unusual for fruit. In addition bananas have some constituents that are also effective for digestive problems: pectin, magnesium, and potassium. Pectin tightens loose bowels, and magnesium and potassium are lost in large quantities in diarrhea and need to be replaced. Pectin is the active ingredient in the most popular brands of over-the-counter diarrhea medicines including Kaopectate.

Another common and popular source of pectin are apples. Apples can be eaten in many forms to give you your dose of pectin, but I would avoid having them in a pie form since that also gives you a lot of fat and sugar along with the pectin. One recommendation is that you grate the pulp and allow it to stand in the air until it turns brown. Because apples are such a good digestive aid you should also include dried apples in your traveling kit when you are driving, and snack on these instead of on potato chips or cookies.

Pears, although they do not contain pectin, have a very soothing effect on the digestive system in attacks of diarrhea. Simply take a couple of pears, removing the seeds and skin, and blend them with a glass of carrot juice, Serve chilled as a digestive aid, and calmer of the stomach. As a preventive you should have a glass of this drink in the morning and in the evening each day.

DISEASE PREVENTION

Disease is easier to prevent than to cure. Just think about it, disease is caused by damage to your body, and getting well is repairing that damage. The more diseases you have the more likely it will be that not everything will repair itself correctly when you get well.

FIGHTING OFF AND PREVENTING DISEASE

Preventing disease largely consists of avoiding doing those things that cause disease. We can often do this by having a diet low in fats and sugars, and high in complex carbohydrates, fruits, and vegetables. While this is a good first step we may still be exposed to infectious agents. Most of the time if our body is well nourished and strong we can resist these infections, and even if we get sick from one of them the sickness is usually short lived.

The Chinese philosophy in fighting off and preventing disease consists of keeping the body always in balance. That is you should get the correct amount of rest and exercise. You should have just the amounts of fruits and vegetables, and of course meats. Whatever you do that might be injurious to your body should be done in great moderation.

In our diets and behaviors it means that you keep your intake of fats, refined flour, sugar, and alcohol to a minimum. Eat fresh fruits and vegetables in season, get plenty of exercise and rest, and keep your mind as well as your body stimulated and alert.

If this advice sounds foreign to you it might do you good to read your Bible, or listen to what the Mormons call the Word of Wisdom. Both of these books ccntain prescriptions for a healthy diet that are very close to what I have just outlined. While the advice may not be specific, it is something that every-one can do, and should do.

HOW TO DISEASE PROOF YOUR BODY FOR A LONGER AND HEALTHIER LIFE

There is a popular natural health magazine that has been around for many years called Prevention, that promotes dietary and behavioral methods of protecting you from disease to give you a longer and healthier life. Now they have printed hundreds of stories and thousands of of pieces of advice on how to accom-plish exactly what we are talking about. I will attempt to sum-marize a little of this wisdom to give you some directions in which to go. Perhaps this will nudge you in the right direction, and you can always go to the source and read all of the stories yourself.

Above all, prevention requires proper nutrition. Nutrition, however, is not a closed and settled field of human health. New information is always being learned, and you have to be a student every day if you are going to get the best possible advice. Consistently appearing in our articles are the benefits of foods high in vitamin C and vitamin E in the diet.

Another large component to disease resistance is attitude. So long as you have a healthy attitude and a positive outlook on life you will have a healthy immune system and be able to resist disease. If you give up hope, for any reason, and give in to despair you will probably be sick within a short time.

Third is to avoid the cures of the medical profession as much as possible. Whenever you can find a natural cure and a natural treatment for a medical or physical problem that you have you have protected yourself from the potential of side effects. There are no numbers on how many people die as a result of their treatments, but it is a good bet that as many die from treatments as die from the diseases they are being treated for.

And fourth, and I will only give you 4 of the hundreds I could give you, is to emphasize fresh fruits and vegetables in your diet. Have them raw whenever possible, and make use of their juice. Do not load your vegetables with butter, cream, or cheese. Find ways to eat them the way they are, atleast do not add as many destructive foods as protective ones. Fruits and vegetables taken in their natural form not only provide your body with the nutrients it needs, but also adds roughage which is good for digestion. Eating fruits and vegetables can be habit forming and keep you away from many ills.

DRY SKIN

Dry skin problems can be caused by wind burn, sun burn, the cold and dryness of winter, allergies, and some diseases. At its worst it can result in sores on any part of the skin, and at its mildest it is still uncomfortable. Most of us develop patches of dry skin, overtime that can be relieved by the use of skin oils or medications, but we can rarely get rid of the problem completely, and it can crop up at any time. In an effort to escape the dry skin blues I would like to give you a list of some foods that can relieve dry skin even if they can't prevent it.

FOODS THAT CAN RELIEVE FLAKY. CRACKED, CALLOUSED AND ITCHY SKIN

Psoriasis, being one of the more serious causes of dry skin, has been the subject of dietary research for some time. A study at the Royal Hallanshire Hospital in Sheffield, England, found that fish oil in the diet effectively healed the flaky, cracked and itchy skin which results from psoriasis. The study used 10 capsules of fish oil a day, but it does suggest that eating fish on a regular basis would also be helpful in healing dry skin.

Going along with the same idea are findings that diets low in saturated fats are also helpful often times in preventing the hard fatty nodules that accompany bad skin conditions. This may be part of the same system that accounts for the effectiveness of fish oil. If the type of fat in our diet affects the condition of our skin, then having a low fat or fish oil diet should be significant. Fish oil, and possibly canola oil, being extremely low in saturated fats, may promote a healthy skin condition.

The skin is naturally oily, but the wrong kind of oils in the diet may serve to block the natural formation of skin oil. The oil on the skin helps to protect us from disease organisms that land on the skin, so that when the skin is dry, sore areas can develop much more easily.

Most foods that help dry skin are used on the outside rather than the inside. A slice of raw potato placed over a dry area will remove irritation and help the skin to heal. It is probably a combination of the starchiness and moisture of the potato that does the job, but its much easier than working out a formula for yourself or buying one at the drug store.

Another topical treatment for the summertime is to use fresh cut strawberries. Just take some strawberries and cut or mash a few up to make a paste, apply to the dry area and leave in place for a while. Finally go to the fruit bowl for a banana the next time you have a dry skin problem. Peel a banana or two and place the soft inside portion of the banana skin next to the dry area. Within a few minutes you should have relief from any discomfort and it should assist healing.

EARACHE

The most common cause of earaches is probably the common cold. With a cold your sinuses run, you blow your nose, and you block the tubes that connect your ears to your sinuses. The result is an earache, and even a possible ear infection. Other illnesses can show up in the ears, although a simple collection of ear wax can eventually block the ears and cause an earache. In extreme cases you can have abscesses, or physical injuries to the eardrum from loud noises. Some swimmers are prone to earaches because they get water in their ears that may be difficult to remove.

Luckily there are a number of household food cures that can be used to relieve earaches. Among those easiest to use are hot onions. Take an onion and bake it, or microwave it, until tender. Then cut into sections and place a few of the warm leaves against the sore ear. Keep the rest of the onion warm, and when the first slice cools replace it with a fresh warm one. Continue this treatment until the earache improves. Onion is said to draw out the pain of the earache.

We usually only think of pumpkins around Halloween, but it may worthwhile to also consider the pumpkin when we have an earache. To cure an earache with pumpkin you need to have access to a pumpkin vine, at least that is what is recommended. Anyway, take the pumpkin vine, slice it and squeeze out some juice. Then place a few drops of the juice in the painful ear and, by reports, the discomfort should clear up within an hour.

The last solution I will give is something that comes from your flower garden. If you are prone to earaches grow lobelia, or buy a tincture of lobelia. If you use the tincture place 6 drops in the painful ear. It works very well on very painful earaches. To use direct from the garden you should make a tea of a few leaves. Then drink a cup slowly as a general pain reliever. It will not work as well as the tincture, but you can use the plant itself as the source of treatment.

ENERGY PROMOTERS

As one of the plagues of modern man most of us are afflicted with low energy levels at different seasons of the year. Older folks develop a chronic low energy problem and could use a pick me up on a daily basis. The rest of us might like a daily use just to avoid those periods when we are just too tired to move.

With these needs in mind I would like to give you some foods to put into your diet that will help you overcome the low energy problem. Give your life more enjoyment by giving yourself more energy.

5 FOODS THAT GIVE YOU MORE ENERGY

Are you a believer in Chinese medicine? I tend to be although I don't understand all of it that well, but I tend to think that a healthy population of one billion people must have some good ideas about medicine. Of course with a population this large they have a lot of older people, and these people are always interested in something they can do for themselves to counteract the typical complain of low energy and vitality. Of course Chinese medicine has listed to this request, and several thousand years ago began to give ginseng to its older citizens, and those with problems of low energy. Not too surprisingly it worked, at least that is what a couple of hundred million Chinese say every year. Now ginseng is available in several forms, but tea is the most common. A lot of Chinese swear by American ginseng, and other countries package it as well, but Korean ginseng is the most common and the cheapest. If you shop around in your local Asian community for a market you should be able to find a ginseng tea for about $7 for 100 packets. Just dissolve it in warm water and drink, sugar may be added if desired. For best effect you have ginseng tea 3 or 4 times at day, spaced at equal intervals.

A food which many avoid, but whose use as a food goes back to Biblical days are beans. Beans have long been associated with being a vitality food in local folklore, although that seems to have been before the days in which its gaseous nature was fully appreciated. Beans are useful as a vitality food perhaps because of their combination of high protein content and high fiber content. In any event, if you are letting a problem of dietary gas prevent you from including beans in your diet regularly there is a drugstore product called Beno that is designed to minimize the gas problem. On the other hand, after a few years on a high fiber diet I have found the gas effects from all of these foods to decrease to a normal level over time.

If you are into fruit and vegetable juices, and still have an energy problem, you are perhaps unusual. When I have used fresh fruit and vegetable juices I have generally had a great feeling of renewed vitality which I attribute to the concentration of vitamins and minerals, along with enzymes, that you get in these drinks. However, one in particular is recommended specifically for energy, and that is carrot juice. The reason is not not known for this effect, but it has been suggested that it is just the sugar content of the carrot juice. I do not fully agree with this conclusion, but I do believe that carrot juice is an energy booster.

One thing I really like in the summer is a vine ripened tomato. In fact they taste so good at that time of year that I will often eat 2 or 3 every day so long as they last. I won't do it with market tomatoes, but the fresh ones really seem to give me a pick up. Well, in my reading I have come upon reports that

Japanese doctors have been prescribing fresh tomato juice to restore the energy levels of people with low blood sugar. It seems that the complex sugars, and other vitamins found in fresh tomatoes have the ability to restore the body's blood sugar to a normal level, and that this is one of the major characteristics of low energy. I am determined to plant a few tomato vines next summer as well just for the energy benefits.

If you love Mexican food I have some more good news in regard to energy. I have already talked about the benefits of beans, but one of the usual spices of Mexican food also serves as an energy booster. Cayenne pepper, added to Spanish rice or refried beans, promotes the energy activity of the central nervous system. This simply means that it will help to wake your mind up, which is a good idea since the heaviness of Mexican food often leaves you feeling heavy and tired. I actually don't recommend a big Mexican meal as a means of getting over your energy blues. They are just too heavy in fats, the way we in America have them, to be a daily part of our diet. But that does not mean that you can't make a nice Mexican style dinner at home, avoiding the fats, and get all of the benefits from the beans and cayenne.

EXCESSIVE WORRY

The old folk song says it takes a worried man to sing a worried song, but excessive worry can destroy you. People worry about all sorts of things, but mainly about things that worry can't fix. They worry whether a relationship will last, when the only way to tell is to wait and see if it does, and they worry if they are overweight, when the only solution is to diet and exercise to lose weight, and they worry if their children will grow up to be good citizens, when you have to wait 20 years to find out. Worry doesn't fix any of the problems that we worry about. That much should be clear.

Most solutions to excessive worry have to do with how we treat life, and I will talk about that a lot, but first I would like to give you a food resource that will help you control excessive worry. This is only a start, but if you combine it with the other suggestions I will give you it should help get over the problems in life that you face.

L-tryptophane is a natural tranquilizer found in all complex carbohydrates. Maybe this is why vegetarians are thought to be passive and meat eaters aggressive. Anyway when you eat carbohydrates, which are found mostly in starchy plant foods, you will get a natural calming effect from a chemical reaction in the brain. If you eat proteins at the same time the calming effect is interfered with. If you are in an anxious mood have a baked potato or a piece of whole grain bread. Stay away from the meats, and do not have any milk products at this time. Within a few minutes you should feel better. By the way, tryptophane is called nature's sleeping pill.

On the behavioral side, and you can't sit around eating potatoes all day long, there are a number of activities you should do instead of just worrying. These are things you have to make up your mind to do, and perhaps you will feel more willing after having some carbohydrates.

To begin with consider the area in which you live. If you live in a crowded city condition you are preconditioned for worry and depression, which are closely related. If this is the setting you are in you need to get out to some open spaces as soon as possible. Do not sit in an apartment or a house alone all day and worry about how bad things are.

Control the sound quality of your living space. If you live in a noisy area play some music to drown it out. Don't just live with it. Studies in the flight path of airports have found depression and disturbance among the people in these areas. If you are used to playing modern, hard rock music, shift to soft music of some sort. It does make a difference.

Now think about the environment in which you feel best. Is it when you are with friends, or when you are alone with a book or some music. If you always feel good in a particular setting this is what you should aim for. It means examining your past life, particularly if you are in a state of excessive worry now. Find the setting that most makes you happy and put yourself into it. Over time it will have a profound effect.

Whatever the setting you live in make sure that you get some fresh air every day. The Carbon Dioxide that builds up in any closed home will depress anyone, and it will not help you if you are already worried about the problems of life. This is especially true if you, or someone in your home smokes. If you smoke don't do it in closed rooms. If someone else in your home smokes get away from them each day for a couple of hours and get some fresh air. It is not just Carbon Dioxide that you are getting, it is Carbon Monoxide, the same thing that comes out of the exhaust of automobiles. How do you think you would feel if you spent every day breathing auto exhaust?

If you have a gas stove in your kitchen, open a window. Gas pilots have two bad habits, they raise the level of Carbon Dioxide, and they release natural gas into your living area that is not burned. The amount in both cases is small, but living with it over years doesn't do you any good. If your stove has an automatic sparker don't worry about it since you don't have an open gas flame anyway.

Just a couple of other suggestions and I will let you out on your own. If you are suffering from excessive worry do something. Become active, because acting is the opposite of worrying about problems and never taking any action. You will be surprised how many problems you can solve by trying to solve them in contrast to how few you solved by just worrying about them.

Finally, take a vacation. Vacations are often criticized because they take you out of your environment without solving any of the problems you left behind, and then return you to it afterwards. However, vacations are a great tonic just because of this process. When you remove yourself from a problem setting you generally stop worrying about it. Instead you worry about the bed you are going to sleep in or if the bathroom will suit you?   In addition, will you be entertained by what you see or do? All of these are very real concerns, but they are also concerns totally separate from those that have caused you worry. This allows you to focus upon the core of the problems that worry you.   If you still can't see a solution to the great problem causing you excessive worry, it probably doesn't have one.

In that case you might as well stay on vacation for as long and as often as you can and let it resolve itself. If you do see a solution then go home and do it. In either case vacations will get you away from the worry and may even give you the solution to your problem.

EXTENDING YOUR LIFE SPAN

We all want to extend our life span, and the trick is simple, just don't die. Well that is too simple. What I really mean is that to extend your life span you have to avoid doing things that are likely to kill you. You would like to know what some of those things are? Of course you would, and there are many answers.

First, we will assume that you have no bad habits. Then what good habits should you have? Follow the old rule of all things in moderation and you will be well on your way to living longer. For instance limit the amount of red meat you have every day, but also limit the number of calories you have in your diet to what you burn up in energy. These two little tips will prevent you from gaining weight and from getting clogged arteries because of cholesterol deposits.

Get some exercise, whether it is just a walk in the afternoon or jogging 10 miles in an hour. Regular exercise is very important for keeping your mind as well as your body healthy. Also get your exercise about every other day, if not more often. If you can't do anything even that strenuous then at least go out in your back yard and do a little gardening several times a week. Everything counts and everything helps.

Eat fresh fruits and vegetables in season. While you don't have to be a vegetarian, everyone should have plenty of fruits and vegetables in their diet. If you eat these foods in season you will be getting the highest possible natural levels of the vitamins and minerals they possess. Along with eating these foods don't neglect to juice them for an added boost, if you have a juicer. Juicers can be purchased for under $40 these days, and they are very efficient and easy to use.

A last little bit of advice I will give you is to have close friends and family members, for man does not live alone. And have plans for the future because nothing helps us to survive from day to day better than having something to look forward to. These two gems actually go hand in hand in that having people close to you will give you someone to plan future events and accomplishments with.

While these may seem like little and simple things, they are. Extending your life is not complicated, its just that it has to be done every day in order to work.

ADD 10 TO 20 YEARS WITH THESE FOODS

Along with avoiding certain foods there are also foods that are widely believed to extend the life span. The use of these I recommend, and you can begin with onions and garlic.

I have already discussed onions and garlic in relation to some other problems, but a study of 8,500 people who had lived over 100 years found that the most common food in their diets were onions and garlic. Since it is known that these foods have many beneficial effects on our bodies it is just possible that putting all of them together adds up to preventing death, and prolonging life. I know that I eat onions and garlic several times a week, and that I suffer from no chronic illnesses. I also have few colds or other minor ailments as well, and it may just be the benefits of the onions are garlic that are responsible.

There have been many studies in medicine that have found free radicals involved in such events are blood clots and cancer. The major killers seem to have a close association with these free radicals, and the only way to counter them effectively is to have a diet high in anti-oxidents. Among the anti-oxidents some of the best are vitamin E and vitamin C. Some of the best sources of these foods are fish oil, or fresh fish, citrus of all kinds, and green vegetables.

The best advice I can give you to add 10 or 20 years to your life is to be a vegetarian at least 2/3 of every day. I do not say this lightly, but because I firmly believe that vegetarians have a healthier diet than most of the rest of us. They have no red meat in their diets, they tend not to be overweight and are never obese, and I doubt if you will find any who smoke and drink heavily. These are probably the major killers in our diet anyway. Smoking, drinking, high fat diets, and foods which make us gain weight.

Smoking kills through all of the kinds of cancer you can think of. Drinking kills through accidents and cirrhosis, and probably contributes to other problems if it is excessive. Fat kills through cancer, heart attacks, and strokes. These are the three major killers of our people. Being overweight and obese kills through heart attacks and strokes as well, but also adds diabetes. Taken together these are a set of diseases and health hazards that you would do well to avoid.

Foods I would recommend? I recommend whole grains, always. I recommend fresh fruits and vegetables in season. If not available than take what is available, but raw and prepare it yourself. I recommend high fiber foods daily, such as corn on the cob, onions, broccoli, carrots, peaches, plums, and whatever else you can find. I also recommend that you stay away from all foods that give you more than 10 grams of fat in a serving, and to keep your fat intake per day under 50 grams. Finally I recommend that you take supplements in vitamin E and vitamin C, at the very least.

All of these recommendations, and this advice might be added to, but it all adds up to the fact that to live for an extra 10 or 20 years you are going to have to take advantage of your lifestyle and of your diet. Good nutrition adds up to a long life, one billion Chinese can't be wrong.

EYE PROBLEMS

I have spent many years as a student, and during the course of my studies it has often been required of me to read many pages. Late night sessions studying, and even all nighters doing term papers have not been uncommon. Of course there are many people other than students that are required to use their eyes more than is good for them. In fact suffering eye strain under such circumstances can threaten your whole future.

Of course eye problems go a a lot farther than just eye strain, although that is probably the most common problem. Infections can also affect the eyes, and deficiencies in nutrition can make the eyes susceptible to all kinds of problems. Getting onto vitamins, vitamin A is anti-night blindness vitamin. But we will get to the wider range of foods for healthy eyes. First I am going to begin with some treatments for eye strain.

EYE STRAIN

Doctors call eye strain conjunctivitis. In plain language this just means that the whites of your eyes are reddened, and watering, and that you might have a discharge from your eyes at night. If you do you will know it because the next morning when you wake up your eyelids may be stuck together, or you may just have some dried material around the corners of your eyes. In any case none of this is dangerous if you take care of it.

Basic nutritional advice is simple, and applies to all eye problems. You need to have sufficient protein in your diet, and you need a high level of vitamin A. Of course you have to keep your liquid levels up as well. It is possible for dehydration to cause your eyes to dry out just as it can cause your body to dry out. You can get relief from the immediate discomfort by taking a fresh cucumber, cutting some slices, and placing 2 fresh slices on your eyes. Cucumber works well as a local pain reliever for other things than the eyes, and you can try it for any thing from bee stings to sun burn.

In addition to these rather broad areas to relieve eye strain there are some direct actions you need to take as well. If the eye strain causes pain you need to cut off most of the use of your eyes. Put yourself into a dimly lighted room, and read and watch TV very little. Getting extra sleep at this time can be helpful.

Keep the oils off of your face. Wash gently around the eyes whenever your skin gets oily or dirty, and dry your face with a soft and clean towel. If your eyes are discharging have something soft around to dry them with as often as necessary, but never rub the area around the eyes to dry them.

For milder cases you should not even have to take these steps. Just don't do anything that causes discomfort. If it hurts stop it. A day or two of rest and keeping things clean should clear up a case of eye strain. If your eye strain persists for a week or more no matter what you do see a doctor. You may have an infection and be in need of an antibiotic.

FOODS THAT FIGHT FOR YOU

I have already said that vitamin A and protein are needed for healthy eyes. Adequate vitamin A helps to keep your eyes from tiring too rapidly, and decreases their sensitivity to glare. The problem with protein is that low protein diets are associated with night blindness. Vitamin A is most abundant in green vegetables, and protein is best from whole grains, fish, and lesser amounts of red meat and eggs.

I am a great believer in herbal teas, even if you don't drink them to get the medicinal effect. For the eyes a strong tea make from catnip has proven useful to relieve the inflammation and swelling you get with allergies. Your clue to the sore eyes being caused by allergies might be that the problem always develops when you go out to cut the grass, or clean the dust out of your garage, or anything that you aren't exposed to on a daily basis. To use the tea make it several times stronger than you normally do for drinking, and let it cool. Then soak a clean towel with the tea and place it on your eyes for about half an hour for relief.

Another excellent and easy cure for sore eyes are potato slices. These are used in the same way that cucumber slices are. For sore and painful eyes take a fresh potato, slice it into thin slices and place one over each eye. Keep then on as long as they are damp, and replace as they dry out. This is an old folk remedy, and probably works because of the combination of dampness and the anti-acid effects of the starch in the potatoes. At any rate it is cheap to use and there is no way that it can hurt you. If it works it can't cost you more than a few pennies to use.

If you look at the old Bugs Bunny cartoons you see plenty of examples of carrots being used for eyesight. This is something you have probably heard about since you were a kid, but nobody ever really told you why. Well I want to tell you why. Carrots contain a good amount of vitamin A, and vitamin A is necessary to prevent deterioration of the retina which can lead to blindness. This disease is called retinitis pigmentosa, and it is very serious if you get it, although it is not proved that vitamin A or carrots can prevent it. However, a low level of vitamin A will result in a sensitivity to bright lights, tiredness of the eyes, and poor daytime vision. Frankly, I think that carrots are a fine preventive of eye problems of several kinds, and I eat them in whole, or as juice, very frequently.

FAST FOOD SECRETS

Fast foods are marketed on the basis of good, fast food, and get filled up cheap. Fast foods certainly do all of those things, but it is the way that they do them that causes problems for your diet. I would like to give you a few pointers on some good diet choices in fast foods, but first I think it would be worthwhile to point out some of the things to avoid.

Fast foods fill you up quickly because they are loaded with fat. Fat gives you that full, satisfied feeling faster than any other food. That is why so many of the fast foods are deep fried. When french fries are deep fried they become saturated with fat. A 100 calorie serving of raw potatoes will become a 400 calorie serving of french fries. And what do you think these deep fried fish sandwiches give you. First off, because they are deep fried they have almost as many calories as red meat of the same weight. But when they are served to you the sandwich also include an oil based dressing and cheese. Chances are pretty good that your average double burger and your average large fish sandwich have about the same calories.

Of course fast foods want to do more than fill you up, they also want to taste good so that you will keep coming back.

The very cheapest flavor enhancers you can get are sugar and salt. All of the main fast food items are served with sugar and salt. In addition to taste the salt also gives you a feeling of thirst, which prompts you to buy their soft drinks. The heaviest sugars are served with the ice cream, but since this is milk based you are not prompted to buy drinks afterward.

On the other hand you can have a fast food meal and avoid most of these traps that they lay for you. Many fast food restaurants serve baked potatoes and salad. Have a salad with a lemon and vinegar dressing, and a baked potato with a minimum amount of dressing, and no cheese or chilly. If you want chicken go to one of the broasted chicken restaurants, and never have deep fried chicken. Tacos as pretty good the way they are, but refried beans often have lard added for flavor. Lard is just another name for animal fat and you should avoid it.

Pizzas are difficult to have in healthy portions, but you can minimize the fat and calories. Do not have extra cheese, and stay away from fatty meats. In point of fact you are better off making your own pizza at home than having one in a restaurant.

These are just a few of the suggestions I could make, but they do show you some of the ways that you can make thoughtful and healthy choices, even at fast food restaurants. You can eat healthy in most any setting, but you have to let your brain help to make choices and not let your stomach do all of the choosing.

WHAT RESTAURANTS DON'T WANT YOU TO KNOW

Restaurants are a different matter from fast food places. For one thing they want you to wait at restaurants. If no one waited they wouldn't be able to sell enough liquor to keep their bars open. Of course they are just as cost conscious as the fast food servers. In many restaurants soups and dressings will have corn starch added as a thickener. If they are really cutting corners you may be getting a bowl of corn starch with a little chicken flavoring instead of chicken soup, and that can happen to a lot of other foods too.

Restaurants also enjoy keeping you at your table for a half hour or so while your dinner is being prepared. During that time they usually have some bread handy to fill you up so that you will think that your expensive meals was very satisfying. They will also try to sell you some alcoholic drinks, which have a very good profit margin for restaurants. If they are real smart they will bake their own bread and serve it to you while you wait. Few people can resist warm fresh bread, and little of it is wasted.

Finally, at the end of your meal a good restaurant will bring around a dessert tray as they serve you your coffee. If the desserts look good enough and they can keep you at your table long enough they can probably make a sale. A couple of desserts can cost about the same amount as one of the dinners they serve, and you won't feel the effects of the calories you don't need until you leave anyway.

Don't fall for these tricks by the restaurants. Know what you are going to them for and don't let them sell you a lot of other items just because the restaurant can make profit out of them. If you like to eat in restaurants find some that you like, and make healthy choices out of their menu items. If you can't find anything on the menu that is healthy and special, then change restaurants.

FATIGUE AND BURN-OUT

Fatigue sets in soon after the summer vacation period. Then comes the holidays, which are frantic, and then several months with few holidays and no vacations. There is fatigue and burn-out. If you ever feel like quitting a job it will probably be in that long stretch from New Years to the 4th of July, before you have begun to look forward to your next vacation.

Fatigue and burn-out have a lot to do with your outlook on life, which is why you may go through the yearly cycle I have just given. It also has to do with a couple of other things as well that can be used to relieve it. The repetition of our lives at certain times of the year, along with responsibility, can both contribute to fatigue and burn-out. But along with the schedule that we live we also go through a cycle of dietary changes through the year that can either contribute to fatigue or alleviate it.

Nutritionists are always telling us that we eat the same way today that we used to when we were all farmers, and spent most of every day in heavy labor. We don't do the labor any longer, but we still eat like we do, and in terms of what we eat the winter is the worst time of year. We eat foods that are too fatty, and we have too much sugar. People drink too much, and they party too hard. All of these foods, stresses, and behaviors add up to creating a setting that leaves everyone tired, fatigued, and contributes to the feeling of burn-out on the job.

But just as foods contribute to fatigue, they can help to change our outlook on life, and our feelings toward the world. Perhaps if I give you a list of some foods that can reduce fatigue and increase your energy, you can largely escape the winter/spring burn-out syndrome. This is a step in how to live life 24 hours a day, 365 days a year.

7 FOODS TO REDUCE FATIGUE AND INCREASE ENERGY

The balance of vitamins and minerals in your diet is often behind fatigue and energy loss. Fatigue and worry are the basis of nutritional fatigue. When you are worried all of the time you upset your body chemistry. This eventually gets transformed into fatigue and exhaustion. Now, while you cannot always resolve the problems that are causing you worry, you can increase the vitamins and minerals that are being exhausted by the condition. This will restore your energy levels and protect you from further fatigue.

The chief culprits are iodine, pantothenic acid, and vitamin A. These nutrients are necessary to keep your hormone and sugar levels in balance. Major foods to supply iodine are fish oils, or fresh fish, and beans. For pantothenic acid you can get a good dose in brown rice or corn. For vitamin A you should eat carrots, yams, and spinach.

FEMALE FERTILITY

Healthy women can become pregnant more easily than unhealthy women. Our bodies are machines that require many kinds of fuel, and getting pregnant is a process that requires a special nutritional balance.

How many women have you known who have been trying for months or years to get pregnant and who still haven't been successful? Every time I am around any group of women who are talking about their children, or the children they want to have, there are several who relate stories of difficulty in getting pregnant. I would estimate that as many as 1 in 3,. or 1 in 4 women have this problem at some time in their lives.

Most of the time these women do not go to a fertility specialist for diagnosis. They just keep trying, and eventually most get pregnant. But what is it about the persistence in trying to become pregnant that overcomes the early problems?

It is easiest to think that successfully becoming pregnant was just the result of combining the egg and sperm at the right time, and that for some unknown reason this simple process was unsuccessful over 20 or 30 months of trying before it worked. Personally I don't think that this is usually the case. I believe that many women have borderline nutritional deficiencies that control their fertility. Women without these deficiencies get pregnant in 2 or 3 months. You all know these women, but you don't think of looking at their diets to see if they are doing something differently than those friends of yours who can't get pregnant.

Nutritionists have studied this problem of who gets pregnant and who doesn't, and they have come up with some ideas which may help you build a fertility diet. It has been found that getting pregnant requires sufficient vitamin C, Zinc, B-complex, and vitamin E.

I will start with a few words about vitamin E. Vitamin E deficiency results in female sterility. Since the effect of a vitamin E deficiency are largely hidden, most of the time you don't even know you have this problem. Vitamin E is found in wheat germ oil and whole wheat. You can also take supplements, but you should begin by getting your vitamin E levels up.

Vitamin C and zinc have not been directly linked to female fertility, but do influence the quality of sperm. If your partner does not have a healthy reproductive system you won't be able to get pregnant. To be on the safe side include vitamin C rich foods in your diet as well as your partners. You don't even have to tell him exactly what you are doing, but citrus and chewable vitamin C should become a part of both of your diets. Zinc can be obtained from whole wheat bread and beans. Low levels of zinc result in a drop in the sperm count, which is not too desirable if you are trying to become pregnant.

B-complex, also available from whole wheat, is necessary for overall health, but is useful during the early stages of pregnancy. Adequate levels of B-complex helps to control the nausea that is so common during the first three months of pregnancy. Keeping your levels high can certainly make the early stages of pregnancy more tolerable.

FOOD POISONING

The worst case of food poisoning I ever had was the result of eating ice cream in Mexico. I had been in Baja for a week, traveling across the peninsula and sampling various foods along the way. However, all the foods I had eaten up to that time had been hot. Milk in Mexico is not refrigerated, they don't have the cold shipment that we do, but is sterilized and sold in cartons. This is fine so long as the cartons aren't opened. But once the cartons are opened and the milk is used to make ice cream it is open to contamination. Now I have no way of knowing what it was that I got with my scoop of ice cream, but it made me sick for a full week before I could get the medication that fixed me up. I suppose I lost a couple of pounds that week, but it was all in pain.

Thinking back I guess I have gotten food poisoning about every couple of years. It is just that most attacks only last for a few hours and I don't think about them much afterwards.

Now I don't like food poisoning very much, and I would much prefer to avoid it. To that end I have compiled a list of 10 common types of food poisoning, and what I can do to avoid them. I thought that it might be worthwhile to share this list so as to provide some relief to the rest of you who have been periodically visited by this discomforting problem. And to add a little urgency to paying some attention to avoidance, some of the big time cases of food poisoning that have gotten into the papers in the last couple of years have resulted in long term illness and death. You can't always avoid it, but you can decrease your chances of suffering from it.

10 COMMON TYPES OF FOOD POISONING AND HOW TO AVOID THEM

(1) One of the most common type of food poisoning we get from eggs. When you buy eggs from the supermarket you have to assume they they are contaminated with salmonella bacteria. Of course eggs have their shells of protection, and if you cook your eggs thoroughly before you eat them they won't make you sick. Heat kills salmonella. However, if you hard boil eggs and take them with you for a picnic don't count on being protected. It is common for hard boiled eggs to be put back into their carton after cooking. This will re-contaminate the shells and over a period of a day or two the eggs will have salmonella in them again. To protect yourself from this type of food poisoning keep your eggs refrigerated, and your hard boiled eggs as well. Eggs prepared other ways should be eaten soon afterwards and refrigerated in the meantime.

(2)   Another frequently encountered type is food poisoning from fresh chicken. The poisoning is from the same bacteria, salmonella, but it is easier to get poisoned from it. Most people will say that they have never gotten food poisoning from chicken, and they are right in a way. usually you get the food poisoning from other foods that you have put on the same surface where you handled the chicken. From the market chickens pretty much all come covered in this bacterial. To avoid food poisoning from it you should cook the chicken thoroughly, but

also wash your hands and all areas in your kitchen completely that you have touched with the raw chicken. If you throw away any raw chicken put it in a covered container, and do the same with any leftovers after your meal.

(3) A cause of food poisoning we see more when we visit poorer countries, but which we may also run into here, is E-coli. This is a bacteria that we all carry in our bodies, and can contaminate any food that is not handled cleanly. The only protection against it is to wash all uncooked foods thoroughly, and cook all meats completely. Ground meats are the biggest risk in the United States, and raw foods and tap water the greatest risk in other countries.

(4) In spite of the claims of the pig growers associations, pork is still contaminated with worms, or trichinosis to be exact. This is the poisoning agent you have always been warned against in pork. These little worms only contaminate a small percentage of pork in this country, but they can be deadly if you get a large enough number of them in a meal. Raw pork should be treated like chicken. When you cook it, always cook it completely, and never eat undercooked pork in any form. Clean all areas where you have prepared pork, and wash your hands well before handling any other food.

(5) Insecticide sprays and fertilizers are used on many of the plant foods we eat. Even though the food and drug people tell us that there is no more than a trace of any of these substances left on the foods in the super market, that is only an average. Nowadays we get foods from all over the country, as well as from Mexico and other parts of the world where they have different standards than we do in regard to what can be put on food while it is growing. I am certain that there are at least traces of everything that is applied when we buy our foods. To protect yourself from trace element contamination from this source wash everything thoroughly, and when you cook it discard the cooking water. It is also best if you discard outer portions of leafy foods.

(6) Fish spoils so rapidly that you would think no one would eat it. However, fish does not have to get to the point of smelling bad before it can make you ill. To avoid poisoning from

fish and shell fish you should use only fresh, or commercially canned fish in your dishes. Fresh fish should have very little fishy odor, if any. The scales on fish should not rub off easily, and for fish the eyes should be clear and not milky. Eat fish well cooked, and do not eat fish that come out of polluted bays.

(7) Often times food poisoning is without a specific cause, but is a reaction to changes in the diet to which local people have become adapted. You run into this type of food poisoning traveling in Europe just as you would in South America or Africa. One way to avoid this problem, and it can ruin a vacation, is to eat only canned foods. Of course this is boring, and there is another solution that is almost as effective. When you travel to a foreign land take along a bottle of Malox type anti-diarrheal medicine. Then before every meal take a swallow. I have known people to travel for 6 weeks in Europe using this method and to escape any digestive upsets.

(8) This one is easy, don't eat the foods in your refrigerator that have grown a fur coat. It is a habit of all of us to keep food around in the refrigerator for too long. Nobody wants to waste food, at least not as long as it might be edible. Of course if the food doesn't smell bad, and you clean it off and cook it real well, you might think that it is safe. Well, it might be and it might not be. Some of the bacteria that grows on food can be just washed off and killed with heat, but other kinds produce poisons that get into the food, and that heat doesn't affect. While it might hurt your conscience a little to throw this stuff out, it will be better for everyone if you do.

(9) Resist the temptation to eat wild berries and fruits you may come across growing on the side of busy highways. While the food itself may be tempting, it is an unavoidable fact that highway departments all over the country use weed killers pretty much everywhere. That nice looking fruit could very well carry a full dose of weed killer.

(10) Finally, short of dying of thirst, do not drink water you find out in the hinterlands of the cities. Sometimes running water, that looks pure, brings back that pioneer feeling of living off the land. But here you run across the same problem as you do with fruits on the side of the road, the government sprays poi-

sons all over our forests and streams to control life forms. In addition flowing water could always be contaminated upstream from animals, or even from human use. The risks are too great to be worthwhile. Water coming out of a ground source might be acceptable, but I would even like that certified by the local Ranger.

FOOD SECRETS FOR WOMEN OVER 40

Women over 40 face several health problems they don't share with men. Only women go through menopause, women are mainly affected by osteoporosis, women are the main victims in breast cancer, and women are the most affected by the collapse of the vertebra in the back giving them a hump.

Most of these problems are diminished or prevented by doctors through various medications they prescribe. On the other hand there are those, and some of them are doctors, who feel that you would be better off if you changed your diet as you got older to protect yourself naturally.

Many of the discomforts of menopause may be relieved naturally by increasing your use of vitamin E, instead of depending on estrogen supplements.   Vitamin E is safe, in its natural form, and estrogen carries some risks. Hot flashes can be largely avoided with the use of 30 I.U. of vitamin E daily. Some of the best sources of vitamin E are wheat germ, sunflower seeds, whole wheat, cabbage, and broccoli.

The usual prescription to avoid osteoporosis is to increase the intake of calcium. Some very good dietary sources of calcium are cheese, sardines, beans, walnuts, and spinach. It is also the fault of increased calcium needs due to the changes your body will undergo in menopause that requires these extra nutrients.

Breast cancer is the one problem that doctors do not even give you a diet or supplements to prevent. They usually tell you to stop smoking, if you do, and cut down on the fat in the diet. These are fine things to do, but you need to work more actively against a disease like breast cancer to give yourself the best chance in life. In addition to taking these steps you need to increase your use of fish and vegetables. This will get you away from the calories and red meat, and vegetables have many nutrients in higher amounts than you find in meats. Of course fat has not vitamin or mineral value, only calories.

These steps in the right direction are worth following if you would live long and be healthy as you grow older. Why grow old at 40 when many woman are healthy and active into their 70s and 80s. You can do it too, if you begin to take care of your health before you develop a fatal or debilitating disease. And even if you are sick already, your best chance to improve and get well is to live right and eat right. Never give up, since that is the only disease that can't be healed.

FOOT PAIN

At the end of the day most of us have painful feet. We may also have corns, bunions, or bruises on our feet, but they all hurt. The most typical picture of a person at home after a hard day has them with their shoes off and their feet propped up on a coffee table. Now let us consider what this has to do with foot pain, and what it can tell us to do about it.

Foot pain in everyday life is caused by two things, for the most part. We often wear shoes that are to small for us, particularly prone to this are women, and just standing around in tight shoes cuts off the circulation and tires the muscles creating pain. If the shoes are not tight the pain will be minimized, and if they are the proper size pain will be reduced even more.

The relief of foot pain can be long term, as when you go out and buy a comfortable pair of shoes that are in your size. Contrary to what anyone may think, shoe sizes change very little as we gain and lose weight, or go from season to season.

It is the short term relief that we can use every day. Propping your feet up does help to restore circulation, but it only does so by getting your feet out of the tight shoes. You can get faster and more complete relief by soaking your feet in warm water. Putting in some salts can also help, and the natural foods advisors have a couple of other suggestions you may want to try. Instead of warm water try soaking your feet in a warm and watery batch of oat meal. Just cook up the meal normally, make it watery, and wait for it to cool sufficiently to put your feet in it comfortably.

There is one other alternative you might also wish to try. Cucumbers have been suggested as a pain reliever for eye strain, and they can also be a pain reliever for foot pain. You will need to take 2 or 3 good sized cucumbers, cut them up and puree them in a blender. Then cool in the refrigerator until you wish to use them. When you wish to revive your feet just put them into a shallow pan and cover them with the cucumber puree. Keep it on your feet for an hour and, by all reports, you will have complete relief and comfort.

FREE RADICALS

Free radicals have become important in slowing down the aging process. Of course you may be asking for an explanation of free radicals that makes sense, as well as some reason as to why they are so dangerous.

First, the human body is made up of atoms and molecules, which are collections of atoms. The molecules are linked together to form cells, which can be very large.

Free radicals are formed when the links between the molecules that form the cells are broken from radiation, or some food or other abuse to our bodies. Breaking a few of these links doesn't kill the cells, and it doesn't kill us, but it does make the cells act in ways that they are not supposed to.

Cells also multiply, and if the multiplying cells have free radicals these also multiply. Now over time these free radicals build up in our bodies it is believed that they can cause our bodies to heal poorly, and our cells to die, and strange things like cancer to grow. The more free radicals that we have floating around the more sickly we are, and the more aged we look and feel.

Therefore, if we can do something to get rid of these free radicals, or at least to prevent their formation, we should stay younger longer and be healthier at all ages. With this goal in mind I would like to give you a few foods that can be used to fight off free radicals.

FOODS TO FIGHT THEM OFF

The key word in fighting free radicals is chelation, which may be done medically in a hospital, or nutritionally with your diet. Doctors are required for medical chelation, using a chemical called EDTA, but I would like to discuss the dietary method that you can use on your own, and that you should have in your diet anyway.

The anti-aging foods repair the free radicals over time, and protect the cells from damage in the meantime. It takes several years with diet, but its worth it.

The active foods in this category are high in vitamin E, vitamin C, selenium, methionine, and some other nutrients. We have already talked about vitamin C foods and vitamin E foods in other sections, and the question becomes which foods combine all of these nutrients for the best doses without eating 20 different foods a day?

You cannot get all three of these nutrients in a single food, but you can get vitamin E and selenium from whole grains, and vitamin C is found in all citrus. Leafy green vegetables contain, in addition to vitamin C, many trace elements including selenium. I do not like to bring this up, because it sounds so simple, but the reason we need to plan our diets to include natural and fresh foods is because too many of us depend on fast foods, and refined foods.

It is possible to go for years without ever eating a piece of fresh fruit or a green other than lettuce. Lettuce is not the best green to have in your diet anyway. It has been bred and refined to the point that it is 98% water, and has as little roughage and nutritional value as possible. By selling lettuce this way it has very little taste of its own, and will taste better with virtually any dressing.

Buy the dark green leafy vegetables. Include cabbage, leeks, and spinach. And never buy white bread, always use whole grain varieties, and make it yourself if you can.

GOUT

Gout was once featured in an old Laural and Hardy comedy. Hardy, the fat one, was being driven around the city with a foot swollen huge, and wrapped in cloth. Each time the foot was bumped, and it was often, Hardy would scream and cry out in pain. This was in the days when gout was believed to be a problem caused by the eating of rich foods, and Mr. Hardy looked like just the person to each such foods.

Now, however, we know better. Gout is caused by crystals of a substance, that is supposed to pass out of our bodies, instead collecting around a joint and causing swelling and pain. The substance is uric acid, and it comes from the foods we eat that contain another substance called purines. As the purines are digested uric acid is produced. The uric acid is supposed to be collected in our urine, where it is then meant to pass out of our body. When this doesn't happen as it is intended, we get gout.

Since gout is the result of foods we eat, and the way we digest them, the cure can also lie in how we put our diet together. We can either avoid eating the foods which end up causing the gout, or we can eat foods that promote the uric acid to pass from our bodies. Depending upon how bad your gout is, you may even want to do both.

FOODS TO EAT FOR RELIEF AND PREVENTION

If you have an attack of gout your first order of business is to find relief. Gout is a difficult problem to treat because it is tied up in a combination of what we eat and how our body digests it. Therefore, I will give you the best advice for relief that I have, and then go into what you can do for prevention.

Almost immediate relief can be achieved by eating cherries. This cure was discovered by a Texan named Ludwig W. Blau, in the midst of a severe attack of gout from which he was unable to get relief. In his case he ate fresh cherries in the evening and the gout decreased by morning. After 10 days of eating only 6 to 8 cherries a day the gout was gone. Furthermore, so long as he kept up the habit of eating 6 cherries each day he did not have an attack. To make this cure even more interesting, he later found that any kind of cherries worked at relieving, and preventing, attacks of gout. You can eat them fresh or canned, sweet or sour.

An alternative, and something that should be combined with the cherry plan, is to consume 3 or more quarts of water each day. This is recommended by doctors, and is meant to work by forcing so much liquid through your body that the uric acid is flushed out rather than building up around the joints.

Although gout is still around as a problem, we don't hear about it quite as much as they may have a few years ago. I believe that is because our modern diet has already eliminated most of the foods with the highest level of nutrients that cause gout. There are just not that many Americans who eat kidney, brains, liver, and anchovies in any large amounts.

However if you have gout, and don't eat these foods than you probably have a diet that has a high level of the lower level causes of gout. In most cases these are thought of as very healthy foods, and more Americans probably have a high level of many of them. The most popular ones in our diets are chicken, meat, beans, seafoods, spinach, and oatmeal. While this reads like a plan for good health, if your body has a problem getting rid of uric acid it can be a prescription for gout.

If you have a case of gout that has been bothering you for some time you are going to have to severely limit the foods in the list just given. In their place you are going to have to put foods like cheese, eggs, fruit, nuts, sugar, and vegetables. Now if you really look around I will bet that you can find a pretty good diet out of the non-gout causing foods that I have just given you.

GUM DISEASE

The most common gum disease, and one from which no one is immune, is receding gums caused by plaque. Plaque is just the remnants of the food we eat that collects around the base of our teeth from day to day. If we let it build up long enough it breeds bacteria, and starts forcing our gums to recede and expose the roots of our teeth. If you let this kind of process go on long enough your teeth will become loose and fall out. Of course the plaque and bacteria will also start cavities at the gum line.

The common advice dentists give is for you to brush after every meal, and to floss every day. At the very least you should brush your teeth in the morning and evening, and floss 2 or 3 times a week. Less than this and you are risking gum disease.

The problem with this program is that you can't always carry it out as you should, and many of us are just forgetful. What is really needed, not as a replacement for the plan that the dentist gives us, but as insurance that even if you do forget once in a while you will still have healthy gums and teeth. That is the sum of what I am going to offer you, a simple method of keeping your gums healthy, even at the dinner table and while you are traveling.

A DAIRY PRODUCT THAT CAN PREVENT IT, WHEN EATEN AFTER MEALS

Every meal ends with a dessert of some sort, but it doesn't have to. If you look at the next dinner menu you see in a restaurant you will see not only the usual cakes, pies, and other sweets, but that you can have fruit and a slice of cheese. This is a common choice available, but not one that most restaurants will push very much since it doesn't give them as much profit.

The key to preventing gum disease at the dinner table is to start eating the fruit and cheese rather than the usual sweets. Both will help keep your teeth clean and remove other food particles that can lead to gum disease.

Oh yes, the dairy product that will help prevent gum disease, that is the cheese part of the fruit and cheese dessert. Even at home end a meal with a slice of hard cheese and you can be confident that your gums are protected. Of course you need to brush and floss in addition, but eat the cheese too. All that you need with a meal is an ounce of cheese.

HAIR PROBLEMS

Hair can be damaged by chemicals, the sun, or a poor diet. Unhealthy, dull, and brittle hair is often a sign of poor general health, and a poor diet. Certainly diet should be looked to before you conclude that you have a fatal disease just because your hair isn't all that you want it to be. Of course your hair may be perfect , but if you have been having any hair problems try the foods suggested here for a month and see if it looks better.

3 FOODS TO THICKEN IT AND MAKE IT SHINE

Hair is made up of protein, although it needs certain vitamins to keep a healthy shine, if your diet doesn't have enough protein your hair will be brittle. While everyone thinks of meat for protein, that is not the only answer. A very good source of protein is unflavored gelatin. Unflavored gelatin avoids the sugar of gelatin desserts, and all that you need is 14 grams a day. This is only about 1/2 ounce a day.

Among the vitamins important to healthy hair are the B vitamins and vitamin E. A convenient source of these is wheat germ. You can eat a bowl of wheat germ each day, or use whole wheat foods for bread and cereal.

There is one other B vitamin called biotin that helps hair to shine with a healthy glow. A good source of biotin is egg yolks. The problem with egg yolks though is that they also have a very high cholesterol level. As an alternative I would suggest the use of 3 or 4 glasses of low fat or non-fat milk each day.

These foods will not only keep your hair shining and healthy, they will also help to keep it from turning gray. While you can have healthy gray hair, the graying process itself is a sign that you need nutritional boosters. Use gelatin, wheat germ, and plenty of milk in your diet for a healthy head of hair.

HEADACHES

Headaches can come as crippling migraines, cluster heads that only stop to start up again, stress headaches, or headaches for no reason that you can think of. While stress headaches are the most common, migraines and cluster headaches probably do the most damage. With a mild headache you can still go to work and function like a normal human being, but with a severe headache you may be too sick to do anything for days at a time.

The common reaction to headaches is to take aspirin to relieve the pain. Usually this helps, but it doesn't remove the cause. If you can control the cause you can prevent the headache in the first place. Prevention is always better than a cure.

Research and observation have found that most headaches are triggered by foods to which we are very sensitive. If you can cut out or control the headache causing foods you can prevent most of your headaches at the source.

I can't tell you exactly which foods might cause your headaches, but I can tell you which one to look out for. It you have frequent headaches, and use one or more of these foods daily, it may be fairly simple to find the culprit. But if you have only rare headaches, then whether you use these foods daily, or only on special occasions, it may be very difficult to find the problem food.

The next time that you are plagued with headaches start cutting out these foods one at a time until the headaches stop. Once they stop you can add the foods back into your diet. You should eventually arrive at the one or two foods, or more, that seem to trigger all of your headache problems.

The foods with the largest number of headache victims

are alcoholic drinks (beer, wine, liquors), chocolate beans, cheese, cured meats such as cold cuts or hot dogs, MSG, and pork). There might be other foods as well, but check out this list before looking at other foods. Each of these foods tend to cause headaches by constricting the blood vessels or increasing the heart rate, thus increasing the blood pressure. Of course you may be more sensitive to one than another, so don't feel that you have to give all of these up for a headache free life.

HEARING LOSS

The greatest cause of hearing loss is noise pollution. When your hearing is attacked repeatedly by loud noises the recovery time becomes greater and greater until sounds at certain levels cannot be heard at all. The first loss is in the high frequency areas, which makes it difficult for the hard of hearing to fully understand speech. This is why someone who has partial hearing loss will often ask you to repeat what you say. They can hear you fine, they just can't hear those parts of your voice that rise and fall to differentiate words. The level of sound that can do damage is not all that high. Sound is measured in decibles, and a level of 120 decibles will produce hearing loss within a few months. You can easily reach this level of sound just by turning your car radio up as loud as you can when you are driving down the street. Do you know anyone who does this? I'll bet that you do since every neighborhood seems to have at least one person who does this regularly.

However, nutrition and diet also play a part in how well we hear. An iodine deficiency will affect the hearing. Iodine deficiency damages the function of the thyroid the most, and there will be many other symptoms. It is unlikely that this kind of deficiency will be first diagnosed because of a hearing loss. If you are concerned though just have a few meals including beans each week, and snack on sunflower seeds.

While you can't stop loud noises from damaging your hearing, you can at least make certain that you have the diet to keep your hearing system as healthy as possible. Vitamin A is very important for hearing, and the best foods for everyone are carrots and broccoli. B complex vitamins are vital and are found in wheat germ. Vitamin C, along with many other things, is also necessary to maintain hearing, and can be found most easily in citrus fruit. You also need the sunshine vitamin, vitamin D, and this can be easily gotten through milk. That is why they call it vitamin D fortified milk. The level of vitamin D has been raised in the milk to prevent disease.

This little outline should be sufficient to get you on the road to nutritional support for your hearing. Don't lose your hearing over a bad diet, and in the meantime turn down your radio and start living in a quieter and calmer environment.

HEART DISEASE

Heart disease kills more Americans each year than all the drugs and all the guns put together. It kills more men than women, and in most cases we cause it ourselves by our diet, lack of exercise, and the stress that we live in.

There is no good reason why heart disease should affect so many of us except that the ideal lifestyle that we live is not healthy. In fact heart disease can even be detected beginning in teenagers today. There is nothing good that I can say about heart disease, except to give you some information on its causes and some of the ways you can protect yourself from its attack, and maybe even reverse the processes that cause it.

WHY IT IS OUR NUMBER 1 KILLER

I have already mentioned weight, diet, and stress as causes of heart disease. Most Americans suffer some degree of heart disease by the age of 60, and the numbers go up as we get older than that. Cancer may be more feared, but many of those who die of cancer have heart disease at the same time.

Heart disease kills so many of us because of the ways in which it works. In the first place you may not even know that you have heart disease until you have a heart attack. That first heart attack alone kills many of us, and it is not preventable without yearly checkups, which most of us do not do.

But supposing you have survived your first heart attack, or you have been diagnosed with heart disease in a physical. Can that protect you from dying from it ? While it can't protect you from dying, it can at least decrease the chance of it happening tomorrow.

Heart disease is usually related to a narrowing of the arteries leading to the heart by cholesterol. As the blood supply to the heart is cut off the heart may increase its pumping rate to move the blood that is needed through the body, or the heart may become enlarged through overwork, or it may just continue as it always has been, but with you on medication or suffering a little pain in the heart or shortness of breath once in a while. In any case as your arteries close down it becomes more and more possible for a bit of cholesterol to break off from the artery wall and plug up the last little hole giving you another heart attack.

Heart disease just makes it probable that you will have life threatening attacks every once in while. The more times that your life is threatened the more likely you are to die. Each attack that is not fatal will weaken your heart, and weaken you. If you do not control or eliminate your heart disease you will eventually have a fatal heart attack, and it can come at any time.

4 FOODS THAT CAN PROTECT YOU AGAINST HEART DISEASE

I would like to tell you a little about alfalfa sprouts, apples, fish, and potatoes. While there are many foods that can protect you against heart disease, these 4 are worth special consideration.

I have chosen alfalfa sprouts because they can be added to so many other things. They can be cooked with other vegetables, or added cold to a salad or sandwich, or even added to spaghetti without anyone even noticing. They do not have a great deal of taste themselves, but that is not necessarily a bad thing. They can even be added to soups, and served with any main dish or salad at a meal. However, I have chosen alfalfa sprouts as a major ingredient to foods that can protect you against heart disease because of their fiber content.

In an animal study at the Cleveland Clinic Foundation in Cleveland, Ohio, it was found that monkeys fed alfalfa in combination with a high cholesterol diet had arteries just as clean as monkeys fed on a purely vegetarian diet. Monkeys fed a high cholesterol diet without the alfalfa sprouts developed blocked arteries, the same as any human might. This strongly suggests that a diet that includes alfalfa as a frequent ingredient will protect you from heart disease even if the rest of your diet contains the normal amounts of fat and cholesterol that American diets tend to have. Therefore, alfalfa sprouts are protective against heart disease.

Now I would like to direct you to apples. Apples are high in a fiber called pectin. Pectin is effective in decreasing the level of cholesterol in the blood, and thereby helps to keep your arteries open. There is advice that you should end each meal with a slice of cheese and an apple, well now you see why this would be a good idea.

Now I don't expect you to have fish for every meal, although you could take fish oil tablets every day. Fish is useful in preventing heart disease because it contains omega-3 acids that prevent the blood from clotting. Other helpful effects found in eating fish are potassium, which serves to maintain blood pressure in a normal range, and its promotion of HDL cholesterol. A useful hint is that most any fish will give you benefit. You might consider preparing your fish in a manner that will not increase your intake of salt, but there are plenty of salt free herbal toppings, as well as lemons, all of which go very well with fish.

I have chosen potatoes as my last recommendation because they are so common in our diet anyway. Before anything else I would like to say that potatoes are important because of their high level of potassium. In fact, a baked 1/2 potato gives you all of the potassium that you need to keep you from a heart attack. I would like to give you a warning though before I go. Potatoes should be eaten baked or microwaved and not boiled or fried. Boiling loses most of the potassium, and frying simply adds hundreds of calories that you don't need. Even when you bake your potatoes you should not eat them drenched in butter and sour cream.

I guess you would like a word as to why potassium is important for a healthy heart. Potassium is one of the most important ingredients in the foods I have recommended. It's main function is to maintain the blood pressure at a normal level. Potassium is also abundant in potatoes and fish, so you don't have to buy supplements or eat exotic foods to get all that you need. If you are low in potassium in your diet it may be the very reason that you have high blood pressure in the first place. If you have any degree of high blood pressure I would certainly increase my level of potassium before doing anything else, and then see what happens. While you should also follow any other recommendations from your doctor, I don't think that any doctor will object to including fish and potatoes in anyone's diet.

VEGETABLES OF CHOICE FOR PREVENTION AND REVERSAL

I have already spoken about the use of potatoes and their protective effect against heart disease, but there are many other vegetables that should also be included in your daily diet for prevention and reversal. Both asparagus and broccoli come to mind immediately. The chief benefit of asparagus is that it is a good fiber vegetable, and that it has none of the negative nutrients that can harm you. Broccoli is much stronger in its protective effects. Broccoli is loaded with potassium, to prevent high blood pressure, and it also provides fiber to control cholesterol in the blood. In addition to broccoli, all vegetables from the cabbage family will give you the same effects. These include green and red cabbage, and brussels sprouts. Personally I don't care for brussels sprouts, although it is the taste I object to, but I enjoy the tastes of all the other major cabbage vegetables.

Peas have not come up before, but they are a good vegetable to keep your heart healthy. Their principle benefits are low sodium, no cholesterol, and a good source of fiber. You can pretty much say the same thing about all vegetable from the pea and bean family. Since the protein these vegetables provide is not delivered in a bath of animal fat it adds nothing to your cholesterol load. I have seen reports by doctors and researchers who state that they have never seen extensive heart disease in vegetarians. Now I can't vouch for that 100%, since most Americans who are vegetarians have not been complete vegetarians all of their lives, but with the ability of some vegetable foods to reverse the effects of high cholesterol diets I think there is good evidence that the more you depend upon plant foods the less chance you will have of developing heart disease.

FOODS THAT STRENGTHEN THE HEART

Strengthening the heart is different from protecting it from the effects of a bad diet, or of trying to recover from a life of too much fat and not enough exercise. American medicine does not think very much about the business of strengthening the systems of our body, but Chinese medicine does. Chinese medicine worries about the strength and health of all of the systems of the body, and has identified herbal medicines that help maintain all of our critical organs. Although these ideas are not as well known as our own natural food and supplement programs, they do offer foods that will do what we want. I have called the offerings of Chinese medicine foods because their diet and medicine use the same plant sources to cure problems that were not prevented with diet.

But all that is beside the point. To get onto foods that strengthen the heart, the 1st recommended is cayenne. This is a rather hot spice that you can buy in the supermarket. It is a general pain reliever, but also benefits the heart and circulation, and prevents heart attack and stroke. While using it as a seasoning may be effective if you have no obvious heart problems, it can be taken by the spoonful when you are aware of any problems affecting your heart or circulation.

The next seasoning, medication, is cumin. We know cumin best as a flavoring for Mexican foods, and it also is available in the supermarket. Cumin is effective in strengthening the heart, and is usually taken along with food for which you wish substantial seasoning.

In closing I would also like to encourage your use of nutmeg. While nutmeg should not be used in large amounts, a daily dose along with your food can protect against heart disease. Because of the character of nutmeg it is probably best taken with fruit, or something sweet. However, if you develop a taste for it in other forms there is no reason that you should not vary the method by which you use it. Because of its potential danger I would suggest limiting your dosage to what you would flavor a dessert or glass of egg nog with.

DIET THAT RELIEVES CHEST PAIN

Chest pain goes under many names including angina and heart disease. Chest pain is a term that can be used to describe any type of pain in the area of the chest or lungs, though for our purposes we are only concerned with its use in relation to the heart. The first thing I would like to say is that chest pain can be a sign of deadly heart disease. If you have chest pain, either before or after an heart attack, see a doctor and follow his advice. Experimenting on your own, even with a beneficial diet, may kill you if the damage to your heart and arteries has reached a critical stage. Only a doctor can tell you how bad it is, and he must do that through examination.

Now that you have seen your doctor and you are being treated for your chest pain, you can look into helping yourself through diet. So long as the foods in your diet don't interfere with the medications you are taking there should be no objection from your doctor.

Improving the circulation to the heart is often all that is necessary to relieve chest pain. In addition to medication you should also increase your intake of vitamin E, vitamin A, B complex, vitamin C, as well as calcium and magnesium. All of these are effective in maintaining a healthy circulation to the heart, and all can be taken as supplements.

For natural sources you can get the benefits of several of these at one time. Stick with grains, vegetables, fish, and fruits.

Of special importance are garlic and onions, although oatmeal, soybeans, and a polyunsaturated oil such as canola should be used for your meals.

It is also possible to make a raw juice drink for the heart. The ingredients are: 10 tablespoons of wheat germ oil

1/2 cup of fresh carrot juice

1/2 cup of fresh squeezed lettuce juice

1 teaspoon of lemon juice

If you blend all of these together for a morning drink you will get all of the vitamins and minerals recommended for a healthy heart, as well as relief from chest pain.

HOW TO LOWER YOUR BLOOD FAT CELLS

The source of heart disease is generally laid at the amount of fat circulating in your blood. It is this fat that is deposited on the walls of the arteries, and which eventually blocks the arteries to cause heart attacks and strokes. In any case there are three basic ways to lower your level of blood fat, and it is best if you use all three.

First, become a vegetarian. While there may be some exceptions, it is mainly the fat we get in meat that raises our blood fat level. This is the first step recommended by many natural food nutritionists, and is the basis of the Pritikin diet plan. The Pritikin people have probably had more experience than anyone else in the world in controlling heart disease through diet, and the basis of everything they do is aimed at lowering fat in the diet to as low a level as possible.

Next, increase your intake of potassium. Potassium works to keep blood pressure normal when you get your diet under control.

Last, exercise at least 3 times a week. Exercise cuts down the level of cholesterol in the blood. While the way this works is not well known, it is known to work for everyone who does it. Your exercise can be as simple as a 30 minute walk every other day, or you can go cycling for 2 hours at a time 3 or

4 times a week. The point is that exercise should make you sweat, and it should make you breathe hard. If it does this and it is sustained long enough it doesn't matter much what you do. A warning though is that you should also warm up very well before undertaking any strenuous exercise. Warming up is not necessary if you are going to walk.

There is one other alternative to cutting all meat out of your diet, increase the amount of fish that you eat. Fish has high levels of omega-3 fatty acids that are protective against heart disease, and will help to decrease blood fat levels.

A 50 MILLIGRAM A DAY FOOD TO CUT YOUR RISK BY 50%

A Harvard medical school study found that 50 mg of beta carotene would lower the risk of heart attack by 50%. Beta carotene has also been proposed as a cancer fighter, and of course it can be taken as a supplement.

However, you can also get an excellent dose of beta carotene through your diet. Beta carotene rich foods include broccoli, cabbage, spinach, and cauliflower. There are many vegetables that are rich in beta carotene, and if you include fresh vegetables in all of your meals you are probably getting more than 50 grams a day right now. But if you are not eating fresh vegetables on a regular basis you should find somewhere to buy beta carotene to use as a supplement.

Beta carotene works by raising your level of vitamin A. Vitamin A is important in protecting many of the body's systems. But besides raising your level of vitamin A, beta carotene is also an anti-oxidant, through which action it may help to prevent the formation of blood clots. At any rate a 50 mg dose of beta carotene is good, cheap prevention of heart attacks.

HEART ATTACK RISK CAN BE LOWERED 36% WITH THESE FOODS

I have already discussed this nutrient in regard to pre-vention of heart disease, but I did not tell you that the Women's Hospital of Boston had found that a high intake could lower our risk of heart attack by 36%. The mysterious nutrient is nothing more than vitamin E. Now while I have already talked of vitamin E a few times I will go ahead and name the major food sources again. Use wheat germ, sunflower seeds, whole wheat, wal-nuts, and corn oil.

Except for wheat germ you are going to have to have much more than a 4 once serving each day to get your thera-peutic dosage. To prevent heart attacks up to 1000 milligrams a day is needed. Personally I do not take that much, but I have seen no warnings in higher levels, and no side effects listed for even much higher doses. My own recommendation is to take a supplement of 500 mg a day, and then have two or more serv-ings of vitamin E foods each day. This will not only ensure that you get a sufficient dose every day, but it will also ensure that you get the benefits of all of the other nutrients that accompany vitamin E in natural foods. While supplements can be invaluable in rounding out a diet, you cannot live on supplements alone. For a healthy life every day you must learn to eat right.

HEART STRENGTHENERS

To get your daily dose of heart strengtheners you can use a diet based on tomato juice, brewer's yeast, citrus juice, and wheat germ oil. Wait a minute, let's just put it into a drink, and you can have it for breakfast. Actually this is not a bad idea. Fresh fruit and vegetable juices contain nearly all of the nutrients of the raw whole forms, and because they can be digested so much faster your nutrient levels will go higher faster than if you ate an equal amount of raw, whole fruits and vegetables.

To make this juice just use:

1/2 cup of tomato juice

1 tablespoon of brewer's yeast powder

1/2 cup of citrus juice (any)

6 tablespoons of wheat germ oil

For best effects you should have a glass at breakfast, during the afternoon, and in the evening after dinner.

HIATAL HERNIA

Hiatal hernia is experienced by almost half of the U.S. population. The symptoms are pretty simple to detect: regurgitation of food from the stomach upwards with an accompanying burning sensation under the breastbone. The causes are more hidden, but it may be significant that while so many Americans suffer from this illness, very few 3rd world people do.

Because of these differences it is probable that the cause lies in some difference in the way we live from the way they live, and because it has to do with digestion it is likely that the area of difference is diet. Most of us have diets rich in fats and refined foods, and poor in whole grains and fiber. People in poorer countries have diets rich in whole grains and vegetables, and poor in fats. They have better digestive systems than we do because their food is better for them, at least in terms of what their body needs for digestion.

Food choices to prevent or relieve hiatal hernia should include whole grains, fruits, and vegetables. Among the fiber foods I would suggest regular helpings of berries of all kinds, pears, melons, cabbage family foods, radishes, onions, potatoes, rice, and whole wheat products. Fiber foods should be eaten with every meal even if you still have too much fat in your diet. They will at least help to lower your blood fat levels which increases the rate at which food moves through your digestive system.

HIGH CHOLESTEROL

Not all cholesterol comes from food. Cholesterol is manufactured in our bodies, and is necessary for us. However, cholesterol is also manufactured in the bodies of other animals, and it is not necessary that we eat them in order to be healthy. The highest cholesterol dose we can get in almost any food is found in egg yolks. While nutritionists now say that you can have as many as 3 or 4 eggs a week without overloading your body with cholesterol, you also have to include the eggs you get in baked goods along with what you prepare yourself.

Of course it is not just the cholesterol in eggs that can give you high cholesterol. If you love red meats and buttered foods, you are probably getting way too much cholesterol for your body to handle efficiently. This forces the cholesterol level of your blood to increase, and you begin getting deposits in your arteries leading to heart and circulatory disease.

It is proven every day that cutting out high cholesterol foods will lower cholesterol levels in the blood. Unfortunately once cholesterol has reached very high levels it may never return to normal, and medications are often used. Diet should not be ignored though. While you are cutting out high cholesterol foods you can also increase high fiber foods as a further means of lowering cholesterol levels. Take a look at the suggestions I have on cholesterol lowering bread and muffins for an activist way to help lower your high cholesterol.

THREE TYPES OF BREAD AND MUFFINS TO LOWER CHOLESTEROL

Breads can be very useful in lowering cholesterol. The best breads are high in fiber and low in fat. Some breads have no fat, or very little fat, although they tend to be a bit hard for most people to use every day. At any rate I will begin with a favorite that always comes to mind when you think about healthy baking products: bran muffins.

Bran muffins have more fat and cholesterol than you might think, although they are still useful since the bran supplies fiber. A 2 1/2 inch bran muffin has only 145 calories, about the same number as in a slice of white bread, 6 grams of fat, and 24 milligrams of cholesterol. If this seems like a lot of cholesterol you should remember that a glass of whole milk has at least 10 times the amount of cholesterol as the bran muffin.

I would also like to recommend whole wheat bread. One slice has only 70 calories and no cholesterol. If you have whole wheat breads do not cover them over with fat rich butter or spreads. Most of the fat we get from eating bread comes from what we put on it, not from the bread itself.

I would also suggest that you discover pita bread. These are breads from north Africa, and can be found in any market these days. Pita bread has no cholesterol, and only 1 gram of fat. Total calories are 165, or just a bit more than you get in a slice of regular bread. If you have pita bread I would also suggest that you discover the uses of vegetable based sandwiches and do not fill up your pita bread with meat.

HYPERTENSION

This is just another name for high blood pressure. When doctors talk about high blood pressure they always call it hypertension, and that is also how medicines are prescribed for treatment. Medical books as well as most articles you will see also call high blood pressure hypertension.

HIGH BLOOD PRESSURE

Now I will talk a little about causes and cures of high blood pressure. This is usually caused by a lifetime of poor health habits. The major causes are smoking, being overweight, eating too much, too much fat in the diet, and too little exercise.

Smoking causes high blood pressure through all of the poisons it puts into the body. For reasons unknown it also causes the arteries to become clogged with cholesterol more rapidly, and whatever the stage of heart disease, it also increases the risk of a heart attack.

Being overweight causes high blood pressure by making the heart work harder to push the blood through all of the extra body tissue, as well as making it harder for you to do any physical activity.

Eating too much causes you to become overweight, but it is also a cause of high blood pressure as well. Large meals make the heart pump harder as well as make you less active. One of the most dangerous things you can do is have a large meal and then lay down and not move afterwards for several hours. If you must eat large meals on occasion, then at least take a half hour walk afterwards to help your digestion along.

Too much fat in the diet loads the blood with cholesterol and makes you gain weight. It also slows digestion,and makes the blood move more sluggishly through the body.

Exercise is a kingpin that too many people ignore. Many studies have found that regular exercise can lower blood pressure. Therefore a lack of exercise can raise your blood pressure from a normal level to a dangerous level that can trigger a heart attack. If you do nothing else walk 1/2 hour every other day and you can lower your blood pressure by 10 points. Its that simple.

FOODS CAN LOWER YOUR BLOOD PRESSURE WITHOUT HARMFUL SIDE EFFECTS

Now that I have told you all of the things that can cause high blood pressure, and some of the steps you can use to make them work in your favor, it is time to give you some advice on foods that can lower your blood pressure without harmful side effects. I have brought up the question of side effects because high blood pressure medications all have harmful side effects. On the other hand most medicinal foods have no harmful side effects, and all that you have to know is which ones to use and how often. The question of how often? I can answer right now--every day, and preferably one or more with each meal. But, on to the foods themselves.

Without going into details I will just say that all of the anti-high blood pressure foods are fruits and vegetables. I think that you should begin your plan to lower your blood pressure by increasing your intake of fruits and vegetables in general. Do this even if you can't remember which specific ones I am recommending, or you can't get them because of the season or the cost.

To lower your blood pressure plan your meals around the vegetables asparagus, beans, celery, garlic, onions, and tomatoes. Surely you can find some use for these in your daily meals.

For fruits stress bananas, currants, kiwi fruit, and mangos. Some fruits like mangos and kiwi, may not be available in your community, but everyone can buy bananas anywhere, and currants (raisins) are sold in a dried form in most markets.

By varying between the vegetables and the fruits you can certainly find at least one of these foods for each of your meals. Furthermore, if you try a little bit you can even make an entire meal of the foods on these lists once or twice a week.

IMMUNE SYSTEM WEAKNESS

The immune system is what our bodies use to fight disease and infection. When we are attacked by these organisms our body sets out to attack and destroy the invaders. We get sicker and sicker so long as the invaders win the battle in our body, and then as our immune system begins to win we begin to get better. Of course recovery may take some time if we have been damaged to any degree, but most of the time it only takes a week or two from the time we are attacked to when we are completely well.

Problems arise when we can't win the battles. This happens with diseases like athlete's foot and cold sores, which become chronic. With these diseases our body just walls them off for periods of time, and then we suffer occasionally when our immune systems are weakened.

The attacks are much more serious when the attacking organisms are able to do a lot of damage. In this case we can get AIDS, develop cancer, catch polio, or get tuberculosis. All dangerous diseases, and some of which we can't recover from.

In any event, prevention is the best medicine, I would like you to strengthen your immune system to prevent any disease, or invader, from setting up a successful attack on your body. Just as eating the wrong foods will weaken your immune system, eating the right ones will strengthen it. You all know people who never seem to get sick and you may wonder why? It is not always easy to see why one person is sick all of the time and another goes through life with very little illness, but I will bet that diet has a lot to do with it. Here is your chance to do some prevention that may put you into the lucky, disease free group and take you out of the unlucky, sick all the time group.

If you have weak immunity it will be easier for you to catch diseases, and more difficult for you to get well from them. Of course there are many factors that influence the strength of your immune system. If you have recently been severely sick, or have had immune suppressive drugs in the treatment of an illness, or are deficient in nutrients you can lower your immunity to the point that you are sick much more of the time than you need to be.

When Americans and Indians came together in the early days it was usually the Americans who had the most diseases. This is not so unusual since Americans lived together much more closely than Indians, and could give each other colds, measles and the flu more easily as well. Anyway, when all of these people were living together and there was an epidemic of measles most of the Americans got red spots and most of the Indians died. The difference was the way the immune systems worked.

Any time that you look at two different cultures of people together the one with the worst diet will die much more often than the healthy and well fed one. A good diet is necessary for a strong immune system, and necessary for a long and healthy life.

Certain foods can strengthen your immune system, just as certain ones can weaken it. If you build your diet around immune system strengtheners rather than weakeners you will have greater overall health.

FIVE FOODS THAT HELP STRENGTHEN YOUR IMMUNE SYSTEM TO FIGHT DISEASE AND ILLNESS

Any presentation of foods to strengthen the immune system must begin with the benefits of ginseng. Ginseng is said, by the Chinese, to help the heart and circulation, and to have generally beneficial effects on the whole body. Studies have found increased effectiveness of the immune system, and many Chinese and other Asians take it daily to prevent the diseases of aging and to give energy. I have already brought up ginseng in other areas, but just to reinforce the information I would like to say that 2 to 3 doses a day are recommended, and I would certainly advise a minimum of 1 dose a day with breakfast. The cost is about 7 cents a dose for Korean ginseng at the best prices available.

The other foods I am going to prescribe are actually food classes, and the theory behind recommending them is to prevent the deficiencies that precede a decline in the immune system. Because the immune system does many things, it needs a high level of some nutrients and trace elements of others to remain healthy. When we are dieting, or sick, or even just as we grow older, we tend to limit our diets more and more until we actually give ourselves malnutrition through our choices. When we do that we leave ourselves open to many more disease than we would if we kept a high level of nutrition at all times. Eventually, without proper nutrition, something will come along that will either cripple us or kill us.

The 1st of the nutritional immune boosters is dark, green vegetables. These give us folate, which keeps the immune system from declining, vitamin B6 to aid in metabolism, and iron to prevent infection.

The next are whole grains, which also provides vitamin B6, but also gives us vitamin E for its anti-oxidation properties and to keep our white blood cell counts high, selenium also for anti-oxidation, and zinc for support of the white blood cells. Just for general information I would like to say that the white blood cells carry the immune system throughout the body. The red blood cells carry the oxygen that keeps the body alive, but do not supply the killer cells that fight infection.

The 3rd are yellow vegetables, such as squash, carrots, and sweet potatoes, for vitamin A. Vitamin A protects the whole function of the immune system as well as protecting against the growth of tumors.

The 4th are cold water fish which provide omega-3 fatty acids which stimulate the growth of white blood cells thus strengthening the immune system.

The 5th are citrus for vitamin C which strengthens the immune system to resist the first assaults of infection in our bodies. The Noble prize winner Linus Pauling dedicated many years of his life to showing how vitamin C helped our bodies to resist disease, and to recover more rapidly when we did get sick. I trust his enthusiasm, along with all of the other information, that vitamin C is important to our immune systems and our health.

IMPOTENCE

Impotence is a common affliction of men, especially men who are older or on medication. It is not a natural condition at any age, but it can have many causes. Getting an erection depends upon a good flow of blood to the penis. If you have any kind of circulatory disease it can result in impotence. Many of the medications that are given for high blood pressure or other serious diseases can also result in impotence. Anxiety, stress, alcoholism, and fatigue probably cause most of the impotence that we experience, so suffering it just once should not be of concern to anyone. The problem with these temporary causes is that some men are so sensitive about their maleness that they lose all self esteem if they suffer from impotence even once. Well, I can't stop you from ever having impotence, but I can help you look into the possibility of preventing and treating it with diet, thus putting you back in control.

CAN IT BE PREVENTED AND TREATED WITH DIET?

The question of diet and impotency depends upon the cause of the problem. Studies of young men have found that supplements of zinc and vitamin B-6 can restore potency within a few months. The function of vitamin B-6 is not well understood in this, but the zinc helps to promote the production of sperm.

As we get older we can suffer impotency from a deficiency of the trace element molybdenum. Convenient sources of this mineral are wheat germ, honey, peas, and soybeans. It would seem wise for older men to switch to honey as a sweetener after the age of 50.

In the list above I gave alcoholism as a source of impotency. Often the only method of curing this form of impotency is to cure it at the source, stop drinking. That should be the first treatment you should try anyway if you drink and are having trouble having sex.

Unfortunately the causes of impotence can be complex, and the cures through diet are limited. Nevertheless I would try these before going for a medical solution. The drugs prescribed for you by your doctor have a greater potential for side effects than any steps you are likely to take through diet.

INDIGESTION

Indigestion is not a great problem with most people, but it is something that virtually everyone has had to deal with at some time or other. The peculiar thing about indigestion is that different foods cause it with different people. While spicy foods are usually involved, for some people it's chili, for others pizza, for others spaghetti. It just seems to be a problem for particular people and particular foods. There are many people in the world who get indigestion from milk and milk products because they can't digest them. In fact most food allergies result in indigestion, along with a lot of other unpleasant events.

Luckily there are a few foods that can help out in preventing indigestion. The numbers of the best ones are not large, but they should be used if you suffer indigestion any more often than once a month. It is better to prevent medical problems than to try to cure them after they have gained a foothold in our bodies and damaged us.

YOU CAN CUT IT OUT WITH GOOD FOODS

The dietary cures for indigestion can be divided into foods and spices. Among the foods there is grapefruit, lettuce, olives, papaya, pineapples, and peaches. Grapefruit, and other citrus, is not eaten whole to cure indigestion. Scrapings are taken off of the peeling and made into a tea or eaten by the spoonful for best effects. Lettuce of any type is effective, but it is not eaten in a salad for indigestion. Take a lettuce leaf and whip it up in a blender, then drink with water. Olives should be taken in the form of olive oil as a cure. About 2 tablespoons is considered a good dose, and you might consider having a salad with your olive oil to make it easier to go down. Papayas and pineapples have enzymes that cures indigestion. Just end your meals with a serving of either one to get things moving. I have saved peaches for last because I love fresh peaches. However for indigestion you are more interested in making a tea from the leaves. For the freshest source grow your own peach tree, otherwise go to a health food store and you will be able to buy a peach leaf tea.

I don't want to forget about the spices though. It is often easier to use the spices then to get the foods when you need them. Common spices, available in your supermarket, are caraway seeds, cinnamon, nutmeg, and black pepper. Caraway seeds can be crushed and used to make a tea, or taken along with your meals as an additive to breads. Cinnamon can be taken very pleasantly to cure indigestion in the form of cinnamon toast. Just make a slice of toast, butter it and put a thin layer of sugar on top, then sprinkle liberally with cinnamon. Nutmeg is very similar to cinnamon in the way you can use it, although I have never heard of anyone making nutmeg bread. I would make it into a tea or add some to any dairy based food. Nutmeg is very potent in its flavor, and it can be self governing so far as dose is concerned. Black pepper has the advantage in that it can be added to just about any food. It is so good that 3 teaspoons are recommended as a preventive of indigestion when traveling in countries where the water supply is suspect. Personally I just use about 1/2 teaspoon in each of my meals and I rarely suffer from indigestion. I certainly believe that a consistent dose of black pepper, or any of these foods and spices, can prevent you from getting indigestion in the first place.

INFECTIONS

In spite of all that we do sometimes we still get infections. When infections are limited to simple cuts and colds they pretty much heal themselves, but when they get serious they often require the help of prescribed medications. In very serious cases they require hospitalization for treatment. It is usually this last bunch of infections that can cripple and kill, and it is these that we want to avoid at all costs.

Now we are exposed to infectious agents all of the time. They float in the air and in the dust of our houses. They are in the soil of our gardens, and even on the doorknobs of the buildings we enter. No matter what we do we come in contact with them every day. Luckily most days they don't hurt us, but unfortunately when they get under our skin or into our bodies through eating or drinking they make us sick.

Our goal is to have a dietary plan that minimizes the chance that those infectious agents that get into our bodies will be successful in making us sick, and there are foods which will do that.

INFECTION FIGHTING FOODS

Some very convenient infection fighting foods are apples, garlic and onions, and honey. I have already discussed garlic, onions, and honey in terms of the immune system, and it is the immune system that fights infection. It does not seem necessary to go over these again as you can read the important parts under immunity.

Apples, however, we have not looked at as yet as an infection fighter. As it turns out the old saying of an apple a day keeps the doctor away has a grain of truth to it. Fresh apple juice, and even apple sauce, have been studied by Canadian doctors as treatment for virus infections, and have been found effective. Apples come in many shapes and sizes, and the best ones for infection fighting have not been identified. But the effectiveness of the usual varieties found in our supermarkets that have been looked at are worth using when you first suspect you have an infection. I haven't mentioned this before, but most of the infections we suffer with from day to day are caused by viruses, and apples seem to work best in fighting viral infections.

INTESTINAL GAS

According to studies at the University of California every person passes gas an average of 14 times a day, so you aren't alone. Of course in public we all hide it as much as possible, and you would swear that most people have never had gas in their lives. Of course it just isn't true, it is something that we all have to deal with every day.

If your gas problems are controllable, and do not cause you embarrassment, you really have to do nothing. It is only if you are passing gas in a more frequent and uncontrollable fashion that you need to look into ways to at least cut down on your gas problem. At least we have some foods that help us control gas, as well as ones that seem to promote it. If you increase the one and decrease the other you should be able to make some progress in controlling your own problem with gas.

The foods that cause gas include apples, beans, broccoli, cabbage, soda, cauliflower, dairy products, onions, radishes, and wheat products. Not all of these are going to cause gas, and it will be your job to find out which ones cause you the greatest problems and cut them out of your diet, or at least to cut down on the amount of them in your meals.

If you eat foods that you know give you gas, there is really no way of avoiding it. However, you don't have to cut all of these foods out if you can find combinations that cut down on gas anyway. I have found that over time my problems with gas have decreased even while eating foods that normally would seem to give me uncontrollable and embarrassing problems initially. So time may help all by itself.

Also the method of preparation may have something to do with it. For instance, refried beans eaten with a traditional Mexican meal rarely give me gas, while boiled beans commonly do. Generally the greater the variety of foods that I eat with any of the gas causing foods in my diet, the less the intestinal gas problem that I suffer. My best advice is to never eat the foods that cause you the greatest problems alone, and to try different methods of preparation for those foods that still give you gas.   Only as a last resort should you cut out a food you value just because it gives you a gas problem.

IRON AND CALCIUM

Iron and calcium are two of the vital minerals needed by the body. Iron is necessary for the red blood cells to carry oxygen. Without sufficient iron in our diet we get anemia, and a form of anemia is even called iron deficiency anemia. Iron deficiency can be caused either by too little iron in the diet, or by an inability to digest the iron that we do ingest. At certain times of our lives, such as in certain diseases or when women are pregnant, the need for iron can greatly increase. If the intake of iron doesn't increase at the same time we develop anemia.

Calcium is needed for the structure of our body. Calcium makes up our bones, teeth, and hair, and there is a constant need to repair these structural systems as they wear out. Without a deficiency of calcium you cannot heal from broken bones normally, your hair will lose its healthy look, and you can develop osteoporosis. Women tend to develop osteoporosis after they go through menopause if they don't take precautions. While it is not true in men, the use women can make of their dietary calcium depends to some degree upon their production of estrogen. When that stops their bones lose calcium and become weak.

WHAT TO PUT IN YOUR TEA TO INCREASE BODY ABSORPTION

It's really very simple, all that you have to do to increase your absorption of calcium and iron is to add lemon to your tea. While lemon isn't the only source, it can be added to tea taken with a meal to make calcium and iron more available for your body.

If you haven't guessed already, what I want to give you along with your regular diet is a dose of vitamin C in your meal. Vitamin C increases absorption, and since you aren't likely to have vitamin C with every meal, if you are a tea drinker you can certainly add lemon to your tea. Perhaps that's why the custom has grown up over the years to serve lemon along with tea. It's not just for taste you see, it's also for the good of your blood and your bones.

IRREGULARITY

I have at times had friends who have had episodes of irregularity. The worst that I can recall followed a trip to Mexico where she no doubt had eaten something contaminated. The nature of her irregularity was such that she would go through periods of constipation followed by days of diarrhea in which everything that she ate would pass through her body within hours. It was so bad that her digestive system became inflamed and painful, and she could find nothing that would digest normally.

Her illness lasted for over a year, and over that time she tried treatment with Chinese medicine as well as every medication that our doctors would prescribe for her. It was so bad that she feared for her life at one time, and when her digestive system did return to normal it took months for all of the symptoms to disappear. This is not something that I want anyone to go through, and I would like to give you a few foods that might help you to stay regular.

NEW STUDY REVEALS FOODS THAT HELP YOU STAY REGULAR

Keeping regular is largely a problem of keeping the proper balance of vitamins, mineral, roughage, and liquid in your body. Of course you must also avoid infections of your digestive tract as well.

A good diet for regularity should be based on complex carbohydrates such as potatoes, rice, or spaghetti. Limit your use of refined carbohydrates such as sugar and white bread.

Meat should be used sparingly. Only 4 ounces a day is recommended by most nutritionists. Too much meat will give you more protein than your body needs, not a good thing in itself, and will give you more fat than you should have, and slow your digestion.

Fresh fruits and vegetables should make up the balance of your solid foods, and some of each should be included in every meal. These will supply most of your vitamins and minerals.

Very limited use should be made of dairy products, baked goods, fried foods of any sort, and snack foods. None of these foods deliver good nutrition with a minimum of calories. All, except some dairy products, have too much salt, fat, sugar, and refined flours.

Liquids are best in the form of water or herbal tea. Coffee should be limited to a couple of cups a day whether you are using regular or non-caffeinated. Milk should be low fat or non-fat, and soda, if you use it, should be diet.

JOINT PAIN

Joint pain, which the doctors call bursitis, becomes more common the older you get. When I was in my teens and twenties I can't ever remember having joint pain. Now, at times, a joint will hurt so much that I can't use it for a day or two at a time. Friends of mine have joint pain that never goes away, and some professional athletes who have retired from their sports have joint pain so bad that they can't walk normally. It is a very common and often crippling problem for which most people do no more than take aspirin and apply heat. Well there are a few more things you can do than that, and one of them is to use a nutritional beverage that can relieve it better than aspirin, and with even fewer side effects.

A BEVERAGE THAT BRINGS RELIEF

For fast and reliable natural joint pain relief take your household turmeric, mix a teaspoonful in juice and drink. Have this in the morning and evening, and you should notice a rapid decrease in pain.

Turmeric fights inflammation and reduces swelling, and has been compared to cortisone in its effectiveness. For additional relief you can mix a thick soup of turmeric with a little lime juice for a paste which can be applied directly to the joint, externally. Joint pain is caused by the swelling from the inflammation of the joint. Once the swelling is controlled, and the inflammation is treated, the pain will go away.

KIDNEY STONES

Kidney stones are very common sources of pain, though not everyone gets them. Chances are ,you know, or have met one or more people who have had kidney stones, and you really cannot see what they have done to get the stones any more than you can see what you have done to avoid them if you haven't been a sufferer yourself.

There are actually many more kidney stones around then there are those who have had pain from them. Unless stones get stuck in a channel for the passage of urine they may be entirely silent. In these cases you can live your entire life with them and never know it.

At their worst kidney stones can destroy your kidneys. This is the most serious consequence of getting them, but it is also the most uncommon one. Most stones can be treated with drugs, or broken up with an ultrasound type machine, and be passed. Others, which are too large will require surgery, but the objective of everyone should be to prevent their formation in the first place. If you don't develop kidney stones you will never have to deal with the problems of treatment, nor with the pain of kidney stone attacks.

PREVENTION AND CURE WITH FOOD

Kidney stones are made up of oxalates and calcium. If you have had stones, or have begun forming them your doctor will probably advise you to cut down your intake of foods containing oxalates and those which are rich in calcium. Of course calcium is necessary for good health, and oxalates are found in many foods that are rich in vitamins and minerals that are also necessary. I have already described calcium rich foods in other entries, but you should know which foods oxalates are found in as well.

Oxalate rich foods are berries of all types, grapes, rhubarb, plums, oranges, asparagus, beans, spinach, tomatoes, nuts, chocolate, and cola drinks. I would certainly look into limiting these foods if I had a problem with kidney stones, but I would also look into adding foods to my diet that might prevent their formation in the first place.

Studies in the British Medical Journal in 1981 reported that doses of magnesium and vitamin B-6 were protective against kidney stones. Magnesium is plentiful in chicken, carrots, bananas, milk, and potatoes. Vitamin B-6 is also plentiful in chicken and carrots, but also in broccoli, and rice. Again, if you eat a varied diet you should not have deficiencies in these foods.

LACTOSE INTOLERANCE

Lactose intolerance is the inability to digest the sugars in milk. When you have lactose intolerance you are unable to eat any milk derived foods. This includes milk, ice cream, cheese, yogurt, and may even extend to baked goods which have been cooked with milk.

When you have lactose intolerance, if you eat one of the milk products you will probably get diarrhea, and may even have more violent reactions. For many people there is no solution except to find milk free forms of the foods you can't eat, and that is usually a satisfactory solution.

The problem with lactose intolerance is not that you can't eat the normal milk products since you can usually find forms of the same foods made from soy, and containing no sugar. Also, even though you have lactose intolerance you may be able to eat limited amounts of some of the foods with milk, you will just have to use trial and error, beginning with small portions, in order to find out which and how much you can eat.

The only real danger is that you may be so efficient at cutting out milk products that you do not get enough calcium in your diet. While you can take calcium supplements, and maybe you should, you can also increase your intake of non-dairy calcium foods. These include sardines, carob, soybeans, almonds, beans, buckwheat, and walnuts. There are others that can be useful as well, and while you should not be alarmed at the prospect of calcium deficiency, you should be aware of it and make alternative calcium rich foods a part of your daily diet.

LEG PAIN

Leg pain is usually related to poor circulation. While it may also be the result of exercise, this kind of pain goes away very quickly. But pain in the legs that is the result of poor circulation will not go away for very long, and can signal dangerous conditions related to heart disease and arthritis.

Varicose veins are another source of leg pain. As the

small veins on the outside of the legs become inoperable your leg muscles ache for the lack of blood and oxygen that they need to live. Without red blood the muscles can't replenish the oxygen they use in making your muscles work.

While there are no sure cures vitamin E has worked successfully for many people. Since vitamin E is an anti-oxidant it is possible that just by keeping the blood from clumping it is able to carry enough extra oxygen to the legs to keep them from becoming painful. Doctors often prescribe aspirin for leg pain, thinking of it as a pain reliever. What they may not even consider is that since aspirin is also an anti-coagulant it may also serve to promote additional blood flow to painful area and relieve pain that is the result of a deficiency of oxygen.

But these are just solutions for supplements. I also wish to give you some vegetables that you can put into your diet to accomplish the same thing.

TWO VEGETABLES THAT CAN RELIEVE THE PAIN QUICKLY

For relief from leg pain I would begin having daily meals of baked or microwaved potatoes and green salad. Both the potatoes and green salad will provide vitamin B-6, and potatoes are very useful for adding potassium to the diet as well. Potassium is a blood pressure manager, and that may also contribute to the relief of leg pain.

LONGEVITY

Longevity just refers to how long we live, and unless we are in poor health pretty much everyone wants to live as long as possible. Of course living a long time is often dependent upon living a healthy life as well. You don't see as many older people with poor health habits as you do younger ones because those are the people who die off from accidents and diseases while they are still young. The older ones are generally those who have taken care of themselves all of their lives. Living well is not a guarantee that you will add years to your life, but living poorly and recklessly is almost a guarantee that you'll have to worry about the health problems you might encounter in old age. But, let's take a look at some foods that can add 10 to 20 years to your life.

OVER 50, FOODS TO ADD 10 TO 20 YEARS TO YOUR LIFE

Longevity isn't something that is easily proven. Those who don't make it die off, and those who live the longest are left to vouch for your advice. In spite of these problems, it is still worthwhile to make some decisions regarding the diet that is best for you. Diet can certainly add 10 to 20 years to your life. The best choices can stop a disease process for many years, or prevent one from occurring, which poor habits in the younger years has gotten you ready for. Just so long as you aren't dying right now you can choose foods to give you those extra years, all that you have to do is to do it.

My first piece of advice is to pack in the high nutrition foods to prevent deficiencies. Too many of us get in a rut by the age of 50 that gives us nutritional deficiencies that we never recognize. Put broccoli, sunflower seeds, beans, fish, melons, and the white meat of chicken in your diet in place of whatever else you may be eating.

Cut down or cut out your use of coffee and alcohol. Coffee speeds up the heart, lowers your body's ability to absorb nutrients, and may increase the level of cholesterol in your blood. Alcohol slows the heart rate along with the reaction time, but is also damaging to the liver if indulged in too much, and always adds empty calories.

Finally, cut down on your indulgence of desserts. By their nature they are high fat and high calorie. At least most of them are. Instead put in an exercise schedule of 1/2 hour at the end of each meal. For every dessert you cut out you can subtract 200 to 500 calories a day from your diet.

FOODS THAT CAN ADD 10, 15, EVEN 20 HEALTHY YEARS TO YOUR LIFE

Of course it isn't just the over 50 year odds who should be concerned about caring for their health so they can live longer. Everyone should look out for themselves all of the time. Adding years to your life is one thing, and even the doctors can do that with their drugs and their machines, but adding healthy years to your life is your job.

To accomplish this wonderful task I believe that everyone should take plenty of liquids every day, and most of them should be water. I am recommending water because alcoholic drinks are bad for your liver and add extra calories, and other drinks tend to add sugar or caffeine. Neither of these you want if you wish to lengthen your life and be healthy.

I would next eat fresh fruit and vegetables in season. This may cut down your choices somewhat, but it would assure you the best prices and the best nutritional value you could get for your money.

Find some alternatives to meat in order to get your protein. With all of the soy products and the various bean combinations around there is no reason that you need to eat meat with every meal to keep a proper protein level in your diet.

Lastly, I would put some of the foods into my diet that many people tend to avoid. They are very useful for long term health. In these I included fish, broccoli, yogurt rather than ice cream for a dessert item, and salads made with cabbage rather than lettuce. I believe that this is an adequate list, if fairly followed, to give you extra years of healthy life. Of course you should stop smoking, if you indulge in that addiction at this time. Drug addiction of any sort is injurious to your health, and will certainly not serve to give you either long life or good health.

LOW SEX DRIVE

Is your sex drive normal? Well, is it at least the same as you remember it 5 years ago? If you have doubts about either of these questions you may have a low sex drive. At any age sex should be an exercise pleasantly anticipated, and engaged in on some regular basis. Some people seem to feel that sex is necessary every day, but these are usually newlyweds. For most of the population sex 2 or 3 times a week is completely normal. Even sex once a week is satisfactory for many people, but if you do not even desire sex more than a few times a year you have a low sex drive, and you need to do something about it. Doctors will prescribe drugs for treatment, but it is often drugs that have caused the problem in the first place. I would prefer to try dietary treatments first, and then let nature take it's course. Change the foods you eat and give it a couple of months before you go to the doctor and you may find that you can cure your- self just by curing your nutrition.

COUNTER IT WITH DIET

A great enemy of a healthy sex drive is overeating. I don't mean just overweight, but overeating all by itself. There are very few people who feel like making love after they have taken in twice the amount of food that they need in a meal. I would suggest that you begin by having your heaviest meal at some other time in the day, and eating lightly in the hours before you would like to have your romantic encounter.

I would also recommend restrictions on alcohol con- sumption. Excess alcohol is known to affect even the very young, and as you become older, if you drink on a regular basis, there is even more chance that your drinking will decrease your interest, as well as ability, to have sexual relations.

Finally, you need vitamin E, and you need increasing amounts as you grow older. Since the production of sperm isn't needed to keep us alive, if you are deficient your body may just cut out producing sperm almost entirely and use it for something else. Incidentally, vitamin E is used by the body to promote the growth of cells, and sex damages a great many cells that require replacement before each encounter. Take care of your body"s needs if you want it to do what you want when you want it.

LUNG CANCER FOR SMOKERS

Smoking definitely causes lung cancer, there is no doubt about that. If you smoke your chance of getting lung cancer will be many times what it would be if you do not smoke.

Now that I have said my piece against smoking, I will say that you can take steps with your nutrition to cut down on the risk of getting lung cancer if you smoke. In fact, the great interest in anti-oxidents over recent years has been fueled by the search for a means to prevent cancer of all types. The rates of cancer in those who do things like smoke are decreased if they have high levels of anti-oxidents in their diets.

While I have already discussed anti-oxidents, I believe that it is worth reminding you of the best anti-oxidents, and of what you should do to put them into your body.

The king of the anti-oxidents has become vitamin E. Supplements of vitamin E are readily available, and I would encourage you to take them if you smoke. In addition you should increase your intake of the high vitamin E foods: wheat germ, sunflower seeds, whole wheat, olive oil, cabbage, and broccoli.

Beta-carotene has also been written about much these days for its anti-oxidant properties. The best foods for beta-carotene are carrots, yams, spinach, squash, broccoli, and apricots.

Vitamin C has many other health effects beyond anti-oxidant properties, but it is good for these as well. Great vitamin C foods are citrus, cabbage, tomatoes, and squash.

"M" IS THE MINERAL

Evidence is accumulating that magnesium is a vital mineral for many of our vital functions. But because so little has been said of it up to this time most of us do not think of it in terms of magnesium being a vital mineral. Of course, when a mineral may have as many benefits as this one, a deficiency in it carries just as many risks.

Because so little has been known about the nutritional benefits of magnesium, there is little information in the dietary literature. If you pick up a copy of Prevention magazine you are not likely to run across information concerning the benefits of magnesium. Even most nutrition books do not discuss it, although some of its uses are recognized.

Magnesium has long been known to be essential to our nervous system, and its functions in the operation of our enzyme systems as well. It is a preventive of heart disease, and is found in bone indicating its function in interacting with dietary calcium so that it doesn't end up causing kidney stones. Low levels of magnesium lead to glucose intolerance, contributing to the development of diabetes, and later to deterioration of vision that is associated with the complications of diabetes.

Magnesium supplements are advisable, although you may be able to use a fortified breakfast drink. In any case you need a daily dose of 400 mg, and it can either be taken in a multi-vitamin form, or as a single supplement.

Because of its multiple functions in our body I would not wait for books to appear which discuss exactly what it can and cannot do. Don't overdose yourself, but get your 400 mg a day in order to get all of the benefits of proper nutrition.

For those of you who prefer your magnesium in your diet, there are a few foods that can provide a sufficient level for prevention. A 4 ounce serving of blackstrap molasses will give you 410 mg, and about 6 ounces of soybeans will give you 400 mg. For oats or brown rice you will have to eat about 12 ounces, and for corn, bananas, cheese, or tuna you will need as much as 3 pounds. Unless you eat the high concentrate foods for magnesium it is not at all unlikely that you could develop a deficiency at some time in your life, and that such a deficiency could last for years. Under these conditions I would still recommend at least a partial dependence upon supplements since you aren't likely to be eating 2 or 3 pounds of a particular food every day. Supplementary vitamins are essential for your general good health.

MALE SEXUAL PERFORMANCE

Male sexual performance has largely been discussed under impotence, but that was in rather general terms. In this section we are going to look at it in terms of testosterone levels. To the thinking of some people all of the problems of society are tied to the level of testosterone in men. It is responsible for wars and crime, and rape and violent sports. Of course it is also largely responsible for the performance of males in sexual relationships. Without a substantial level of testosterone males cannot perform sexually.

Unfortunately for this vital function of testosterone, in relation to mental health, testosterone levels are sensitive to disturbances from many sources. Levels commonly decrease with age, but also with the taking of many drugs, and with certain diets. While we can't alter our age, and oftentimes we have to take drugs to stay alive and functional, we can control the major decisions of our diets by some simple planning.

The first step is to find out what foods lower our cholesterol levels in the same way that aging and drugs lower it. Then, just by avoiding those foods, it has been found possible to keep our testerone levels 30% higher.

A DIET TO AVOID, IT LOWERS TESTOSTERONE BY 30%

It is easier to give you a diet to avoid in order to keep your testosterone levels high then it is to give you one to boost it up if it has gotten low. But this is advice for those of you who like a nice dinner featuring lots of meat and potatoes. This is a sure route to low levels of testosterone. Studies have found that following a large meal, especially if it is heavy in fat, testosterone levels will drop by as much as 30%.

When you eat your body devotes its energy to digesting your meal. The more fat in your meal the harder your body has to work to digest it. When you have a typical American meal that is 20% or more of fat, your body devotes extra energy to digest it. As a consequence your testosterone level will drop by 30%.

One more suggestion before departing this topic. If you are having trouble with performance, and you drink alcohol, cut out the alcohol. Alcohol is a depressant and decreases the flow of blood. Since blood flow is a big part of sexual performance, alcohol makes it more difficult to have sex. And while a little alcohol seems to increase the interest in sex, larger amounts act as depressants and decrease it. Therefore, the more alcohol you drink the harder it will be to have sexual relations, and the less interested in them you will be. Furthermore, if you drink in excess the longer you do this the greater the effect on you, in terms of being capable of having sex.

MEMORY LOSS AND COMPREHENSION

Loss of memory is not necessarily a sign of Alzheimer's disease. Preoccupation with problems can cause stress and a temporary loss of memory. Medications and alcohol use can also affect memory. Physical injuries to the head may interfere with recall and comprehension, and deficiencies of diet may have profound effects.

In this book I am most concerned with those causes of disability that can be cured through diet. I can't cure Alzheimer's disease with diet, but I might be able to help sharpen your memory with the proper choice of foods. The better your diet the more likely you are to have a mind that is working at its peak, and the more easily you will be able to comprehend the problems that come your way in life.

FOODS THAT HELP YOU THINK AND REMEMBER

Memory is very sensitive to the balance of certain vitamins and minerals. Those which have shown the greatest effects on memory are vitamin B-1, vitamin B-12, choline, magnesium, and iodine. Vitamin B-1 controls the ability to recall stored memories. Vitamin B-12 and choline are involved in both memory loss and comprehension. Magnesium is involved in the ability to learn and comprehend, and iodine assists the thyroid to function properly. Poor thyroid function is another cause of memory loss. Now I want to give you 7 foods that will cover all of these nutrients at as high a level as possible.

The first food I will recommend is wheat germ. A 4 ounce serving of wheat germ will give you 2 mg of vitamin B-1, 400 mg of choline, and 320 mg of magnesium.

Next I would say that you should get your recommended allowance of eggs each week. Eggs supply 0.32 mg of vitamin B-1. 0.0020 mg of vitamin B-12, and 1700 mg of choline.

Thirdly, fish should be a standard part of your weekly diet. In various fish of different types are found all of these 5 vitamin nutrients.

Fourth, soybeans. It is lucky that soybeans are an adequate protein substitute for red meat since it also contains so many of the nutrients that we need. Soybeans supply vitamin B-1, choline, magnesium, and iodine.

Fifth we turn to cheeses. Cheese is a source of vitamin B-12, magnesium and iodine.

Sixth I would recommend beans. Beans are another protein alternate which can also supply vitamin B-1, and iodine.

Seventh, and last, put nuts into your diet. I am somewhat reluctant regarding nuts since they tend to be so high in fat, but they are nevertheless excellent in terms of memory support. Nuts are good for vitamin B-1, magnesium, and iodine.

METABOLISM MANAGERS AND WEIGHT LOSS

While many people blame poor metabolism for being overweight, it is usually poor eating habits that are usually to blame. Of course this does not mean that metabolism is not an important factor in weight loss, it is just that it is rarely the most important factor.

Metabolism is sensitive to how active we are, and what demands we are making on our bodies. If we do nothing but lay around all day the only energy we burn is the the minimum amount to keep our bodily functions operating. In most people this is less than 1500 calories a day. Moderately active people, like most males, actually need about 2000 calories a day to maintain weight, and not to gain it. Women have different systems of body function, and a moderately active woman will only need 1800 calories. If you are very active, or are a competer in a sporting event, or just a laborer who works physically every day, your needs may be 1000 calories higher.

Of special importance in using exercise to increase metabolism, and gain the benefits of a higher metabolic rate, is that you do it regularly. It is much more valuable for you to exercise twice a week all year around than to exercise 5 days a week through the summer and then not at all through the rest of the year. You will not only keep your body in better condition, but you will keep your metabolic rate at a more uniformly higher level all year. A big problem with exercising is the startup period anyway. This is the time that everything hurts the most, and when you are in the greatest danger of getting hurt, or even of brining on a heart attack. Exercise regularly even if it is not at the level that is recommended. If you have a good start you can always increase what you are doing.

The problem with our weight is that it is just too easy to get too many calories. A full meal at any of our fast food places will give us around 2000 calories. If we have dinner or lunch this way, then even a light breakfast or tea will make us gain weight instead of lose it.

But with all of this said, it is still of interest to try to find foods that will increase our metabolism to the point that we can have an extra 200 calories or so a day and still lose weight.

Foods can help out in lowering weight by increasing our metabolism somewhat, and that is precisely what I want to present. Three foods that can speed metabolism and help you with faster weight loss.

THREE FOODS TO SPEED METABOLISM FOR FASTER WEIGHT LOSS

There are some foods which make your body operate at a higher level than normally. After all, if you are overweight it is often difficult to see where you eat more than those who are thinner than you, or why they are able to lose weight so much more easily.

The first food I would suggest is celery. Many nutritionists feel that it takes more energy to digest celery than you get in it. If you are going to snack, then snack on celery.

There are two ways of going about changing your metabolism through diet. One is to go on a high protein, low carbohydrate diet, and the other is to use a low protein, high carbohydrate diet. Neither of these diets should be used for more than a week at a time since extended used can be dangerous and lead to deficiencies. Nevertheless, if you want a quick loss of 5 or 10 pounds you can use one of these food plans. Just get off of it after a couple of weeks, and wait at least a month before you go on it again.

For the high protein form, use a low fat source of protein, and cut out all carbohydrate, or at least cut it down to just a few ounces a day. Every meal should have fish or lean chicken. Have no high fat foods such as red meat, and all other foods taken in should be fat free.

To go the other way you want to have a high carbohydrate, low fat food. Spaghetti or potatoes are acceptable, just so long as you have them without oils or fats of any other sort. Do not eat beans or soybeans as substitutes for meat, at least for the 2 weeks you are on this diet. You can eat as much of the carbohydrate as you want, but that is all you can have.

MIRACLE FOOD FOR PAIN, CHRONIC FATIGUE, DEPRESSION, AND SLEEPING PROBLEMS

While it may not be obvious, all of these problems are related to your blood sugar level. When the blood sugar level gets either too high or too low it causes disturbances in your body . In terms of Chinese medicine your body is out of balance with either the active forces or the inactive forces dominating the body and producing illness. The proper cure is to use a medicine that restores balance, and cures the problem at its root.

The supreme Chinese medicine for restoring and maintaining balance in the body is ginseng. Ginseng will help to raise the blood sugar if it is too low, and will work to lower it if it is too high.

If you have developed one of the problems listed above you should visit a Chinese practitioner, or a holistic Western doctor for treatment and monitoring since Chinese medicine are usually given in combinations that must be continually adjusted to match the symptoms of the patient.

But if you do not have a disability right now, and would like to prevent one in the future, you can make ginseng part of your diet. I have already discussed the cost and dose in other areas of this book, but I will still remind you that the cost is only about 7 cents a dose, and you should take two or three doses a day.

The Chinese have sworn by ginseng for over 2,000 years, and I have used it with success at various times myself. While ginseng could be a part of everyone's diet, it should certainly be part of your diet if you are concerned about depression or chronic fatigue.

There is one caution I should mention, do not use ginseng if you are suffering from an inflammatory disease, that is one that produces a fever.

MIGRAINE HEADACHES

If you have never had one then you don't know what they feel like, but if you have ever had one you will never forget it. As the migraine comes on your hands get cold, a feeling of fatigue and depression comes over you, lights begin flashing in your head, and your head begins to throb. Shortly the pain in your head settles down to an ache, and you may develop a queasy stomach leading up to vomiting and diarrhea. Fortunately for men this is not one of those areas where men and women are equal; women by far suffer in greater numbers than men.

The triggers that bring on migraines are so varied that if you are susceptible there is no way avoiding all of the goods and conditions in life that can cause an attack. However, among the foods one of the biggest offenders is MSG, which is still used as a flavor booster in many Chinese restaurants. If you have ever had a migraine headache avoid all MSG.

Now I said that there are many other causes as well. There are so many that you can come into contact with them at any time. Therefore, the spice I am going to suggest should be used daily as well. Luckily it is pleasant, and can be used as a tea as well as added to many foods.

Peppermint is the plant, and I will give you a word or two about its background. Peppermint belongs to a family of folk remedies for headache called feverfew. Feverfew is the form recommended in the natural health literature, but peppermint is recommended as an alternate which is cheaper and easier to get, and which has the same effect.

As a spice peppermint can be added to both desserts and meats. It can be mixed into pretty much any foods that are cooked, but most of you may prefer to take it as a tea.

A good formula for peppermint tea calls for bringing 2 cups of water to a boil, remove the water from the heat and add 2 tablespoons of mint leaves. The mint can be either fresh or dried. You want a good strong cup of tea so let the mixture steep for 1 hour, and drink 1 to 2 cups of the cold tea. Take the tea whenever you feel a headache coming on. For extra relief rub tea on your temples and around the back of your neck.

MOOD ELEVATORS

If you suffer from chronic depression, or even just from mood swings that leave you feeling in the dumps for a day or two at a time you would probably like some safe foods you could use to raise your spirits to a comfortable level.

Moods have been found to be very sensitive to vitamin B deficiencies, to low calcium, and to result from certain allergies. B vitamins can be taken as supplements, or you can take whole grains.

If you have ever had a warm glass of milk to calm yourself down before going to sleep you have used calcium to smooth the nerve ways connecting the mind, nerves, and muscles of your body. Bringing the body into coordination allows you to relax completely, and will elevate your mood if you are depressed, or calm you if you are in an excited state.

Allergies are trickier to treat if they are the cause of your depression. Of course you would like to get rid of the allergies, or to remove the substances you are allergic to from your body. Of course if you don't know what you are allergic to it is hard to remove it or avoid it. Therefore, with allergies, you have to take some general steps in the meantime to avoid the depression that comes with some allergy attacks.

You can work to keep your blood sugar level constant by breaking your meals into a half dozen snacks during the day instead of three large meals. This will overcome some of the effects of allergies even if it won't remove the allergies themselves.

The choice of foods, best to accomplish this blood sugar level constancy, is complex carbohydrates such are spaghetti and whole grains. It is not at all uncommon for mood swings to occur in the period between meals as your blood sugar level shifts, and this diet will avoid that.

MOTION SICKNESS

As I was growing up I lived near a cousin with whom I would occasionally have the privilege of going on car rides. Now we did not do that many things together, even as children, but I remember those car rides for the attacks of motion sickness she would suffer. My family would like to go into the mountains at times, and about 10 minutes into the winding hills and we would have to take a stop so that that she could go to the edge of parking area and try to get her stomach under control.

This set of adventures went on for a number of years, although eventually she began taking medication for it, dramamine I think, and gradually got it under control. Still, even though the dramamine controlled the motion sickness I was never comfortable with the idea that you had to take a drug just to take a ride in a car without throwing up. That is why I was so interested when I ran across information about a household spice that can do the same thing, and without a visit to the doctor or pharmacist.

A SPICE THAT CAN PREVENT IT, AND RID YOU OF NAUSEA

A folk remedy long given to women for morning sickness is ginger root. Originally a couple of teaspoons were given directly to prevent morning sickness, although today you can get it in capsule form as a supplement.

Now so far as I have been able to determine the effective agent in ginger is found in the pods as well as in the root, and I have found comparative studies by Bringham Young University in Utah comparing ginger, ginger root, and dramamine for their effects on controlling nausea. They used a spinning chair to test the effectiveness of the various remedies, but I thought that was sufficient.

In any case the ginger products proved to be even more effective than the dramamine in controlling nausea.

So for the control of nausea, in motion sickness, or

morning sickness, take a couple of teaspoons full of ginger. If you cant get that much down then purchase ginger root capsules and use the equivalent whenever you are going into a situation that is expected to produce nausea.

MUSCLE SORENESS AND PAINS

Muscle soreness and pain can be the result of exercise, and that is fully expected if you get a lot of physical exercise, but sometimes it develops from injury or disease.

Going on a hike one time I rotated by shoulder to slip a pack frame on my back. At the end of the hike, about 3 hours later, I found my shoulder to be a little stiff. I put it down initially to the strain of the hike, but it didn't go away in a day or two like I thought it would. Instead it got worse and worse, and for nearly 3 months I barely had use of that arm and shoulder.

Following an Xray, that found calcium deposits in the shoulder, and a months worth of therapy, the pain finally went away. Over this period I would have given a lot for a diet that could have relieved some of the pain without all of the drugs and therapy that I ended up taking. Let's see what I have come up with that might help you.

DE-TOXIFYING FOODS THAT CAN END PAINFUL MUSCLE CRAMPS

Even though calcium deposits are often the cause of muscle pain, calcium is just as often the solution as well. If you have a problem with chronic muscle pain and cramps increase the calcium in your diet through the use of non-fat milk and cottage cheese. Calcium tablets can also be used if you would like a supplement.

If the calcium alone is not as effective as you would wish then add an 800 I.U. dose of vitamin E to your diet. Vitamin E promotes healing, and it is just possible that your muscle pain is lasting for a long time because you are re-injuring the same muscles each day. Vitamin E will help speed recovery and healing.

Vitamin D has also been promoted as a muscle pain reliever. This is where double duty comes in. If you are drinking milk to get calcium, milk is also fortified with vitamin D, and you will get your dose of that at the same time.

MUSCLE TONE

Good muscle tone is the result of exercise and a good diet. If you have a sound diet, and you exercise regularly there is no reason that you can't continue to have a good strong body all of your life. Contrary to the belief of the too young, your body does not fall apart after the age of 40. Actually it can fall apart at any time that you quit using it. If you get too lazy to walk a mile or do your own yard work you are also probably too lazy to get out and exercise as well. These are the little old people of 40 or 50 that you see walking around who are incapable of doing anything active any more.

Luckily the days in which this was an ideal life style are pretty much past. Today no one is thought to be incapable of going out and finding a sport or bit of exercise that they can do to maintain muscle tone. After all, how long has it been since exercise gurus have been promoting walking as a means of getting in shape. Not too long ago you would be told that if all you did was walk, you might as well do nothing at all.

Now that the attitudes toward what constitutes good exercise have changed so much, it is time to look back to the diet end of the muscles to find the nutrition that you need to stay in shape.

But, in the belief that it is harder to keep a well toned body the older you get, we will look at foods or the over 40 person, that will help shape and tone the body. If they work in the middle aged person they will certainly work for anyone younger as well.

SEVEN FOOD SECRETS THAT HELP YOU GET BACK IN SHAPE AFTER 40

Go for the foods that give the benefits of high nutrition and low fat. Broccoli provides vitamin A, vitamin C, and calcium; sunflower seeds provide vitamin B-6 , folate and iron; beans provide vitamin B-6, folate, magnesium, and iron; salmon and the white meat of chicken provide vitamin B-6 and folate; and cantaloupe provides vitamin A and vitamin C.

I have chosen this list of foods because studies have found that 1/3 of those over 40 are not getting enough vitamin A, vitamin B-6, calcium, and magnesium in their diet. About the same numbers come up for shortages in vitamin C, folate, and iron.

If you want a lean body , with good muscle tone, at any age you have to reduce your calories, reduce fat, increase essential vitamins and minerals, and increase roughage.

OSTEOPOROSIS

When women go through menopause and their estrogen production declines, their bones begin to lose calcium. As the bones lose calcium they weaken. In fact they weaken to the point to where the vertebra collapse, making some women into hunchbacks, and just leaving others susceptible to broken bones from such things as turning over in bed in advanced cases.

Osteoporosis is a silent disease in its early stages. Even though most older people develop it to some degree, and some are crippled by it, before it starts causing pain you will probably not even know that you have it. That makes it all the more important to concentrate on prevention, if prevention is possible. I believe that it is, and in a minute I will give you some ways to go about it.

While women may be at greater risk of osteoporosis than men, it is not usually recognized that lighter skinned people are more at risk than darker skinned ones. This indicates that the threat of developing this disease is something that we are born with, and not something that is totally controlled by diet or behavior.

Traditional treatments for osteoporosis have been to give women estrogen supplements, and a diet that is high in calcium in the hope that osteoporosis can be stopped or avoided all together.

An interesting study by the Pritikin Institute in Santa Monica, California, found a correlation between diets high in animal proteins and imbalances in calcium, magnesium, and zinc. One of the results of this imbalance is a high level of osteoporosis. The imbalance was noted in diets that were as little as 25% animal protein, and the effects occurred in men as well as in women, even with calcium supplements as high as 1400 mg.

Well you are just as able as your doctor to chose foods that will help strengthen the bones. While it is a complicated problem that can't be cured by just a few foods in the diet, at least you can get a head start on controlling osteoporosis.

FOODS THAT STRENGTHEN BRITTLE BONES

While it is necessary to maintain a high level of calcium at any age, especially for women, it becomes even more important once a woman has hit her 40s. A good, anti-osteoporosis diet, should contain 1000 mg of calcium, but also a high level of phosphorus, and low fat.

For breakfast use toast, juice, and milk. Limit caffeine drinks. For lunch have a carbohydrate food such as pasta, broccoli, and milk again. You can make up a vegetable snack, or use non-fat yogurt if you like. Dinner should be fish, a green vegetable, rice or potato, milk, and a fresh fruit for dessert.

As you can see, this first day's diet minimizes foods you shouldn't have, and boosts those that are high in the nutrients that you need.

Controlling osteoporosis also means controlling your intake of caffeine. Caffeine speeds up the rate that calcium is taken from the bones. To counteract the effects of caffeine you can increase your intake of magnesium. Magnesium has already been encountered in regard to many other health benefits. Besides all of the other less common sources of magnesium, bananas are certainly one of the easiest ones to include in your daily diet. In addition to bananas I would also like to promote that you alternate with apples. Apples supply boron, and boron has been found to stop the loss of calcium from the bones.

In addition to diet, even a mild degree of exercise increase the calcium content of the bones. As you eat a good diet, also take regular aerobic exercise.

AN EVERY OTHER DAY DRINK THAT CAN PREVENT OSTEOPOROSIS

Do you like a glass of wine every now and then, or some other alcoholic drink. There has been a lot of publicity lately about wine preventing heart attacks, but nothing about the relationship of alcohol to osteoporosis. There is a relationship, at least for women. Alcoholic drinks raise the estrogen level in women. This helps a great deal in preventing osteoporosis since it is the drop in estrogen at menopause that is believed to be the main cause of the disease. There are cautions however. Only one drink every other day is necessary in order to get the health benefits. If you drink more than that you are doing it for some other benefit than disease prevention.

If you don't drink, don't start. There are alternatives to using alcohol for the prevention of heart attacks and osteoporosis, but if you do then manage it. Since neither of these helpful effects require more than one drink every other day. This amount should help you without hurting you in any way.

OVERWEIGHT

It is not exactly a simple question to ask if someone is overweight or not. Undoubtedly most of the American population feels that they are overweight since most of them are trying to lose weight all of the time. If you feel that you would just like to lose 10 or 20 pounds, or maybe even more, you have lots of company.

Of course our diet and affluence don't help either. We have quite a lot of money, at least most of us do, and food is relatively cheap. Many of us live at fast food restaurants where they want to give you something satisfying and filling for a few dollars, and that is what you want too. It is any wonder that fast food places put as much fat into their foods as they can get away with. Fat only costs a few cents a pound, and if used just right you never taste it. If you really want to get an idea of the fat in one of these meals just buy one and let it get cold. The fries become stiff with grease as it cools, and the burgers become unappetizing and stiff as well. Unless you buy a diet type meal, you might be getting half of your calories from fat in these meals.

But back to the problem of being overweight. There are plenty of tables around to tell you if you are overweight or not, although you probably know exactly how you stand on that anyway. Most of us have a target weight that we think would be just right for us, even though we may have never actually weighed that amount.

In the name of helping you attain your target weight I will give you a list of 12 foods that actually consume more calories in digestion than they give you when you eat them. This can be the start of a diet based on something other than low calories and exercise.

NEGATIVE CALORIE FOODS THAT FORCE YOUR BODY TO LOSE WEIGHT

Naturally negative calorie foods are largely made up of water, and most have very little nutritional value. After all, proteins and carbohydrates have calories as well as fat, just not as many. On the plus side, even though they may not have high nutritional value, they can supply a lot of roughage to your diet. Since our diets are usually low in roughage this is a very positive feature of negative calorie foods. Roughage doesn't count against you because it is left largely in tact as it passes through your digestive system.

Some foods that are mainly water and roughage include alfalfa sprouts, asparagus, bean sprouts, berries, cabbage, cauliflower, celery, greens, leeks, lettuce, and tangerines. If you eat these foods without added butter, and microwaved, steamed in water, or raw, it is impossible for you to gain weight, You would have to eat so many pounds of these to gain weight, alone or in combination, that you simply cannot hold that much.

Just because these foods are mostly water and roughage do not think that they have nothing else to offer. While they do not have proteins or carbohydrates in any significant amounts, they do provide a high level of certain vitamins and minerals. Sprouts are high in vitamins A, C, E, and B-complex. Cabbage is proposed as a cancer fighter, and tangerines are an excellent source of vitamin C.

This is typical of the negative calorie foods. It will be difficult to obtain a filling diet based on these foods, but if you use them for snacks and incorporate them into each of your meals you will not only help yourself lose weight, but you will keep your vitamin and mineral levels high.

PERFECT FOODS THAT CAN BE VERY BAD FOR YOUR HEALTH

Some foods are called perfect because they provide all of the required vitamins and minerals, as established by the government nutritionists. However, just because these foods can prevent you from getting deficiency diseases, it doesn't mean that they do not have things bad for your health.

One of the perfect foods is eggs. Eggs provide complete protein, as well as all of the vitamins and minerals that you

require. The egg yolks also provide a high level of fat and cholesterol. If you eat whole eggs you should limit yourself to no
more than 4 eggs a week. If you just eat the yolks you can pretty much eat what you want, but you are no longer getting a perfect food. The white of the egg is mainly protein, and the yolk
carries most of the vitamins and minerals that make it a perfect
food.

Milk is another perfect food. A glass of milk, especially
when it is fortified with vitamin D, has all of the basic proteins,
vitamins, and minerals that you need. If it is a glass of whole
milk it also contains much more fat than you need in your diet.
If you depend on skim milk you will avoid the fat, but you still
won't get the roughage that you need.

I would advise you not to look for single perfect foods.
Diet, nutrition, and health are best taken care of through a wide
variety of foods. You should have a diet that mixes 100 different
foods each month, or even each week. If you go any 2 days
without varying your diet you are in danger of developing a deficiency disease.

You also have to take care to get a wide variety of foods,
and of particular types, when you are sick or have special
needs. If you are healing from an accident or operation you will
need more calcium and vitamin C than you would otherwise. If
you have a problem with high blood pressure your need for
potassium will be higher than otherwise. If you are depending
upon a perfect food to supply all of your nutrition needs you are
in definite danger of missing out on special nutritional needs that
may develop at any time. People change from day to day, and
your needs for diet do to.

PAIN RELIEF

You can have many different sources of pain. Sore muscles are painful, but usually only for short periods of time.
Fevers cause bodyache, but that disappears when the fever
goes down. Injuries cause pain, and it can be of long or short
term duration, and vary from severe to almost too mild to notice.

Illness can also cause pain, and sometimes pain management from illness becomes more important than treating the illness itself.

I have never had a pain that was severe for more than a few days from any source, but I have a cousin that has had chronic lower back pains for most of her life. It has been so bad that she has had two spinal operations, including a fusion of her lower spine, which required a full year to heal each time. The pity of it is that neither of these operations cured the problems, or the pain, with her back. Just because a doctor says that a course of treatment is the best thing for your pain, don't accept their word until you have looked into it yourself.

There are a series of steps you should take yourself before you let doctor's do their act on your painful body. To begin with most pain will go away by itself if you wait long enough and don't injure the part of the body that is affected. In the meantime you can try aspirin or Tylenol, which all of the doctors recommend for mild pain any way, and alternating heat and cold.

If these first cures are not effective within a few days, you will have to decide for yourself exactly how much, you may be in need of stronger treatment. No one should suffer chronic pain without doing something about it. Personally I hardly ever take medication for pain, but when I do, I make careful judgements as to what I take and how often.

But before you go to your doctor for medication to relieve pain, with all of its possible side effects, there are safer cures based upon diet which are nearly as effective, and which do not have the problem of side effects or cost that prescriptions get into.

OINTMENTS WHICH WORK FAST AND ARE LONG LASTING

The newest rage in the health community is an ointment made from chilies called capsaicin. When taken internally it is very hot, and takes some getting used to, but when rubbed onto areas of sore muscles it is very effective and long lasting. It used to be available only in health food stores, but as it has gotten more popular it can often be found selling over the counter in local pharmacies.

Turmeric is a spice that can be purchased in the supermarket, but which has very effective pain relieving properties for bruises and other muscle injuries. Just take a tablespoon and mix with enough water to make an ointment. Apply the ointment directly to the injured area. Turmeric can also be combined with other pain relieving herbs or spices to vary its effects.

Wild mustard growing throughout the country offers a convenient and free source of an ointment with a long history of use for pain. Just take the fresh leaves of mustard and crush them into a pulp. Spread Vaseline over the painful area of the body, apply the pulp on top, cover it with gauze and tape it in place. This mustard plaster can be left in place for several hours, and the Vaseline will prevent the skin from blistering.

Finally, a quick relief from the pain of burns and sunburns is pumpkin. Simple canned or fresh pumpkin applied over the painful area directly from the refrigerator works almost instantly. This is an old prescription from the Navajo Indians of Arizona who have been growing pumpkins for hundreds of years, and have had just as long to figure out uses other than carving them into faces or making pies out of them.

NATURE'S MIRACLE PAIN RELIEF FOODS

I have already mentioned the use of peppers as an ointment for the relief of pain. Eating meals flavored with chili peppers will supply the same substance internally. It is useful against virtually all forms of pain, and can be taken as often as needed.

Generally pain can be helped by drinking large amounts of liquids, preferably those that calm you such as warm milk or tea. Stay away from the heavy protein foods like red meat.

Onions or garlic, or some other high fiber foods may be the best choice if the pain is in your digestive system. Do not resort to alcohol for pain relief, and go lightly on all caffeine foods including coffee, chocolate, and cola drinks.

For a high dose of vitamins, minerals, and fiber use dried fruits such as figs, grapes, apricots, and prunes. Because of their condensed form eating small amounts of them during the day can keep your nutrition levels high.

AN EFFECTIVE, LONG LASTING RELIEF THAT'S PROBABLY IN YOUR REFRIGERATOR NOW

Those of us who enjoy Mexican foods always have a little jar of cumin in our refrigerators. What we don't realize when we are making those wonderful dishes is that cumin is also useful as a pain reliever. Depending on how it is used it can relieve the pain of liver problems, as well as stomach and gall bladder pains. A tea can also be used for muscle spasms.

To make the tea pour 2 cups of water over 1 teaspoon of cumin seeds, and let steep for 1 hour. Then just drink the cold tea at the end of the hour to relieve the muscle spasms.

Other uses require making a poultice of 2 and 1/2 tablespoons of cumin seeds by soaking them in hot water, strain and dry them thoroughly, crush them, and mix with a little white flour and water. Use just enough water to form a paste, apply to the stomach, and cover with a light towel or gauze bandage.

PMS DISCOMFORT

PMS discomfort varies from woman to woman. Most women do not even have PMS, but of those who do some have claimed that it has been responsible for them murdering their husbands and children. This very extreme reaction to a natural process in womens' bodies makes it important enough that an attempt should be made to manage it in all women that it bothers.

If you have PMS, and have resorted to over the counter, or even prescribed medications to decrease symptoms maybe it is time to give some natural remedies a chance. Wouldn't it be pleasant if you could just change your diet a little bit for one week a month to get rid of it. PMS is common enough that there should be a simple, safe, and natural method of dealing with it, and that is what I would like to give you here. No single remedy will work for everyone, but if these foods relieve the symptoms for at least some of you than they are worth while.

5 PROVEN PMS RELIEF FOODS

The foods suggested are based on the relief given for PMS by vitamin E, and that vitamin B-6 needs to be present, but in small doses. Sometimes PMS is caused by thyroid problems or low blood sugar, so it is also important to manage these areas to have the best chance of curing the symptoms.

The food highest in vitamin E is wheat germ. Wheat germ can be purchased inexpensively by bulk, and used either as an additive in other foods, or directly to make a cereal or mush. Wheat germ also has a modest amount of vitamin B-6, but it should be enough to help relieve the PMS and not enough to produce side effects.

While it only has a fraction of the amount of vitamin E that is found in wheat germ, whole wheat still has a sufficient amount to be effective. The value in whole wheat is that it can be found in all baked goods, and is available pretty much anywhere that you buy food. The vitamin B-6 levels are about 3 times what is found in wheat germ, but again there should be no problem with a side effect. I would recommended that you go entirely to a whole wheat diet at least a week before the schedules beginning of your period.

Since thyroid function has sometimes been involved with causing PMS symptoms, it is only appropriate that you protect yourself with foods that strengthen thyroid function rather than weaken it. Vitamin D is one of the most important nutrients to thyroid function, and for that I recommend cold water fish such as sardines, salmon, or tuna. These foods do not supply the other essential vitamins for thyroid function, but some of these are found in the foods already listed for PMS relief.

If you are not getting extra vitamin B-6 brown rice should be included to relieve PMS. Brown rice has one of the highest levels of B-6 of any of the foods you might use for a main dish, and is the only one of which that you might eat in servings of more than 4 ounces.

A 5th food which should be excellent for PMS relief is rose hips for vitamin C. Vitamin C has been found very effective in both preventing PMS and is ensuring a rapid recovery for symptoms. Alternatives might be to just increase your use of citrus fruits in the week you generally experience problems.

POLLUTANTS

Pollutants are a growing threat to your health. Once upon a time you could go into the mountains or desert, or away from the cities into the country and escape the pollutants that city people had to suffer with. That time is no more. Pollutants are killing the trees in the forest and have added smog to the deserts. The county has all of the malls and trucks of the cities, but has added poisons for insects and weeds, as well as fertilizers for the crops grown.

Our homes aren't even safe any more. If you use even half of the chemicals recommended by markets for household cleaning, your home is constantly full of fumes. And our food now comes with pesticide residues, and is made with altered genes to make them grow faster and not spoil. There is almost nothing you can do that does not expose you to pollutants.

Luckily for us our bodies can resist most of the pollutants we are exposed to. Unless we breathe them in or eat them they usually just land on the outside of our skin and clothing and can be removed by washing. Ones that are strong enough to effect us through our skin need to be taken away as soon as possible since they can hurt us rapidly and badly.

The pollutants we breath are pretty much out of our hands so far as ridding our body. But the pollutants we get with our food, and which pass through our digestive system, can be protected against and removed from our body without harming us if we take the proper steps. I will give you a few ideas of how you can start getting rid of the pollutants in your body.

RID YOUR BODY OF ENVIRONMENTAL POLLUTANTS

To remove environmental pollutants you should start with the outside of your body. I have already noted that you can simply bathe to remove pollutants from your skin, and that most won't get below your skin anyway. Of course if you have any breaks in your skin or weakness in your immune system you will be more susceptible to pollutants from the air, and even from your home and clothing attacking you through your skin. As a consequence I recommend more than just bathing. At least once, and preferably 3 or 4 times a week take enough exercise to work up a good sweat. This will open your pores and flush out the surface layers of your skin. As an alternative you can take a good sweat bath every other day, or as a last resort use a good, hot tea. Drink enough of it to make yourself sweat. Then bathe and clean your skin completely. Staying clean through bathing will take care of most of the pollution you will be exposed to.

For pollutants that you take into your body, they will either go to your digestive system or into your respiratory system. You can protect your digestive system by having a diet high in fibers and low in fats. However, for extra protection you can use some natural remedies at least once a week to flush out your system. Olive oil is an excellent detoxicant for your digestion. It promotes the pancreas to increase the amount of digestive enzymes, and it helps the ball bladder to release more bile.

It is very hard to remove pollutants from your lungs once they have gotten down there. But at least you can take nutrients to protect yourself from their effects. The protective nutrients for the lungs are vitamin E, vitamin C, and vitamin A. These can be taken as supplements, or you can include wheat germ, citrus, and fish in your diet to boost your nutritional intake. This would be a good idea even if you did not know it, your lungs had been exposed to pollutants or not, just as a preventive of negative health effects.

PREVENTION

This whole book is about prevention more than it is about cure.   Foods can heal, drugs can heal, and exercise and life style can heal. But I am more interested in what can be done to prevent illness, and I want to tell you why I believe that preventing illness is better than trying to cure it.

WHY AN ONCE OF PREVENTION IS ALWAYS BETTER THAN A POUND OF CURE

Every doctor will tell you that it is 10 times easier to prevent an illness than to cure one. Even a simple illness means discomfort, but it is usually not possible to prevent these anyway. The simple illnesses you are likely to get are colds and athletes foot.

Somewhat more serious illnesses are usually not dangerous, but can be under certain circumstances. These can be prevented in most cases, and the reason that they aren't is that people are either too lazy or not interested. These include the flu, measles, and mumps. For some people these illnesses can lead to birth defects, or complications can easily put you into the hospital.

More serious diseases are more difficult to prevent, but the consequences of getting them can be very dangerous. These include diabetes, high blood pressure, arthritis, and heart disease. Prevention is a life long process in which you have to eat right and exercise, as well as watch your weight from day to day and week to week. Once you have acquired one of these diseases you usually have to live with it the rest of your life even if it doesn't kill you.

The most serious diseases are also the most difficult to prevent since the causes are only partially known, and your risks of getting them often increase with age. These include cancer, heart attacks, strokes, and AIDS.   These can all kill you.

Prevention is necessary for a long and healthy life, but if you are like most people you will be suffering from more than one of these in your later years. I probably should not include AIDS in this group since the causes and risks are much better known, but it is an incurable disease that kills and for that reason is put with the others.

Prevention will not only save you a lot of pain and disability, it will also give you the ability to feel good and be active and in control of your life whether you live 60 years or 90 years. Ofcourse, poor health is expensive as well, so saving money by not preventing illnesses costs you a lot more money when you do get sick both in getting cured or treated as well as in lost earnings. I can think of nothing good to say about behaving in ways that end up getting you sick when you have the option of preventing the sickness in the first place.

PROSTATE CANCER

Prostate cancer is a disease of men, and usually of older men. Most men, after the age of 50, experience an enlargement of their prostate. Sometimes this enlargement is a sign of cancer, and only a doctor can tell for sure. In the early stages prostate cancer has no symptoms, and so progresses to the point that it becomes deadly. There is a debate as to whether men should be treated at all for prostate cancer once they have gotten into their 70s or 80s, but that debate has not been settled. At this time if you get prostate cancer you face surgeries, radiation, and chemo-therapy. Because most of these cases are not caught early on these treatments just cause a lot of discomfort and do not cure the patients. They are looked on as the only chance for most men though. It is also unfortunate that treatment for prostate cancer also ends the sexual relations of most of the men who undergo them, but that is inevitable with what is done. Luckily you can take some precautions to decrease your chances of getting prostate cancer, and perhaps save yourself from becoming one of the 34,000 yearly deaths it causes.

FOODS THAT PROTECT YOU FROM ITS 34,000 YEAR-LY DEATHS

To protect yourself from prostate cancer you should start no later than the age of 50, and ideally by the age of 40. Certainly by this time you will be able to make your own decisions as to which foods to eat and in which combinations.

Animal fats are known to be a risk factor in many cancers, and prostate cancer is not exception. You need to stop using oils with saturated fats and cholesterol and emphasize vegetable oils and fish. Those most strongly associated with low prostate cancer rates are olive oil and canola oil. In countries where olive oil is used predominantly there are lower rates of prostate cancer, breast cancer, ovarian cancer, and colon cancer. Olive oil also promotes efficient digestion, something that saturated fats do not do, and canola oil is even lower in saturated fats than olive oil. Canola oil has the advantage that it is much less expensive than olive oil, although it does not have the same qualities of taste. For effectiveness either one is excellent. For cost canola oil is far cheaper, and for taste and as a digestive aid olive oil is superior.

Experimental studies have been performed on prostate cancer using powdered beet root. Although this may not be a standard treatment for cancer as yet, the studies found that the beet root had the ability to break up cancer tumors. This would seem to indicate that a regular diet which included beets could be preventive of prostate cancer. In the studies the beet powder had a very strong effect, but had no side effects. You may have to be creative in finding recipes for beets that will fit into your lifestyle, but a regular serving of beets in some form each week may well be worth the effort.

Beta-carotene has more recently been introduced as a cancer fighter. In its natural form it is found in carrots, and in large enough quantities to be effective against prostate cancer. So far as what carotene is in itself, it is just a form of vitamin A, of which carrots are known to have large amounts. A preventive dose of carotene for prostate cancer is 12,000 IU, or 2-/2 times what the government recommends for a minimum daily requirement. Carrots, in raw and shredded form, will provide 31,000 IU per cup, and in cooked form 38,000 IU per cup. Carotene is one nutrient that is not destroyed in cooking.

PROSTATE PROBLEMS

Other then cancer, the prostate offers other problems which are not uncommon, and which must be treated when they occur. A simple enlargement of the prostate, without cancer, will still restrict the flow of urine and cause great pain. It often must be treated by cathertization by a doctor.

Enlargement of the prostate and pain may also be the result of prostatitis, or inflammation of the prostate. When this is a result of infection you may need antibiotics for treatment.

In all cases the best course is to avoid developing prostate problems in the first place, rather than trying to figure out how to cure them once they start causing you pain. Let's look at some of the ways to avoid them.

WHAT TO DO TO AVOID THEM

Prostate infections may be prevented with a tonic which is used to treat them after they have developed. Taking the tonic this way is using it in the same way that you might use a birth control device to prevent pregnancy. If you are boosting your immunity at the time you are exposed to an infectious agent you are much less likely to get the infection in the first place.

You may be able to find the prostate tonic in a health food store, but if you can't you can probably find the ingredients. Here is what you need: gravel root, uva ursi, parsley root, goldenseal root, cayenne, juniper berries, and marshmallow root, all in equal amounts; and 1/2 of the amount of each of the others for licorice. These will all be dry ingredients. You just mix them together completely. A dose is 1/2 a teaspoon taken 2 times daily either dry, or in warm water as you would a tea.

For prostatitis you can make a tea out of a combination of herbs similar to the one above, but with a few variations. Mix equal parts of gravel root, uva ursi, echinacea, parsley root, and ginger root, with 1/2 part of lobelia. Put 2 ounces of this mixture in quart of water to make 4 cups, and use this amount each day.

Another preventive of prostate problems is made from ginger root. Ginger root is available in the supermarket, and the prescription is to use it externally. Take 1 whole ginger root and grate it by hand. Put the grated ginger root into a piece of muslin or cloth that can be tied tightly closed and place into water boiling on the stove. Leave it there for 7 minutes. Then remove the root and use the tea for warm compresses in the area of the groin and anus, front and back. If you are actually suffering from prostate problems at the time use these compresses for 45 minutes at a time, and once every 4 to 6 hours. For preventive use weekly, single application of 45 minutes should be sufficient.

PSORIASIS

This skin condition is more embarrassing than painful or dangerous. It is also limited somewhat by age. If you are over 40 you are unlikely to develop a case, but between the ages of 10 and 40 it can show up at any time.   Causes are many, being anything from a poor diet, to an infection, to just going through some kind of stress such as taking a test or losing some money.

There are no precise cures although some of the ways studied for dealing with it include the removal of foods like wheat and oats from the diet. This was studied in France and many of the patients did get better. In some people meat and eggs seem to be the cause, and all of this supports the idea that psoriasis is not just one disease, but is just one of the common symptoms of food allergy.

IT CAN BE CURED BY SOMETHING FROM YOUR HEALTH FOOD STORE

Health food stores earn their names. Of course you can get something from your health food store to cure psoriasis. One of the recommended cures, according to the alternative medical community, is lecithin. You should even be able to buy lecithin in bulk in some health food stores, and all that you have to do is take at least 4 tablespoons a day for up to five months.

I have given you these numbers because in a study of 254 psoriasis sufferers found that 4 to 8 tablespoons taken for 5 months cured all of them. This doesn't mean that you can't use less and be cured more quickly, or that if you take more you will be cured more quickly either. It just takes time to cure psoriasis.

If you want to get your lecithin in food form rather than in supplements the highest lecithin levels are found in wheat germ, nuts, seeds, whole grains, and vegetable oils.

SEXUAL PERFORMANCE

Sexual performance varies for men and women. A woman's interest in sex may affect her performance, but women can fake it much more easily than men. It is only when a woman loses interest in sex to the point that she won't even fake it that her performance suffers. Of course a woman with a genuine interest and enjoyment of sex will usually be a much better sex partner than any other kind, but it is not always possible for a man to tell the difference.

Of course when you talk about sexual performance you are usually talking about men. A man cannot fake an erection, nor can he fake an orgasm. A woman can roll around, tighten her muscles, and heave her body, and men won't know the difference. But if a man does the same thing, and doesn't have an orgasm, a woman can tell it every time.

Sexual performance in men is very emotional as well as physical. If a man has a companion in whom he is not interested for some reason, he may not be able to perform. How his partner looks is not usually the deciding factor, although men are not generally attracted to women who are very much overweight.

Much more important than looks though is the psychological problem of compatibility. If you fight with your spouse constantly, and are usually in a state of anger, you are unlikely to become very much aroused when the chance for sex does arise. Consequently poor sexual performance often follows an unhappy social situation.

Other, more physical, factors affecting sexual performance are your health, your nutritional levels, drugs you may be taking, whether or not you drink, and how much, and even age to some degree.   Age certainly affects sexual performance, but very elderly men are capable of a very satisfying degree of sexual performance even if they don't perform in the same way as a man of 30.

Alcohol, in regular and substantial amounts, will have a very profound effect on sexual performance. If you drink regularly, even small amounts, and are having trouble with sex, cut out the drinking. While you may be able to just cut down and do fine, unless you cut it out all together and find out if drinking is the problem you won't be able to judge what you can tolerate and maintain a healthy interest and function in sex.

Drugs are a greater problem. If they are just recreational drugs, you can cut those out too. But if what you are taking is for an illness you may not have that option. Because drugs for cancer or heart disease must be continued, you should consult your doctor about possible courses of action that might restore your sexual function to a level you would like to have it.

Baring these various causes we are still left with nutrition. A vitamin deficiency can also affect sexual performance, and the only way you can detect such an effect is to add foods or supplements that will strengthen sexual performance. Poor nutrition can cause a decreased blood flow to the penis inhibiting your ability to get an erection.

This kind of blood flow problem is cured with a process called chelation which removes tiny clots from the vessels of the penis. the main chelating foods are bananas, kiwi, mangoes, and papaya. These all have a high content of chelating minerals and an enzyme called bormelain, which has some chelating affects as well. A banana a day may do more than keep the doctor away, it may also help you have a little fun at the end of the day as well.

SHINGLES

Shingles is an extremely painful condition in which a red rash forms around part of the trunk of the body, and is accompanied by extreme pain. It is called a neuralgic pain because it is caused by inflammation of the nerves. It usually occurs sometime in midlife, in the area of the waist or chest, and while the discomfort usually goes away in a few months, oftentimes the rash may go away and leave the pain. Then the pain may persist for additional months or even years.

The doctors offer pain killers, or may even offer surgery in extreme cases, where they propose to go in and cut the nerves that are causing the pain. But pain killers can fail as you become accustomed to them, and surgery is permanent while shingles is not. It is only because the pain is so extreme that anyone should consider it.

However, it may help to give you some more information about the cause of shingles, and how it can be treated naturally. I always prefer to use natural treatments if they are available, and this is true whether or not I am seeing a doctor at the time or not. Doctors will always take credit for cures, though they may blame your home cures for their failures if their drugs don't work. Don't let that bother you though, after all, it's your body and your decision as to how to take care of it.

WHAT CAUSES IT AND WHAT YOU CAN DO ABOUT IT

Shingles is caused by the same virus that causes chicken pox. In fact if you have ever had chicken pox you are carrying the virus around in your body, and it can develop into a painful case of shingles at any time. The way it works is that after you have had your case of chicken pox the virus hides out in the nerves around the spine. Then when you experience a lapse in your immune system due to an illness, poor diet, or stress it attacks your body and you end up with shingles. At least that is the theory after looking at a lot of people and what they were doing when their cases of shingles developed.

Now that you know you have the virus, what can you do about it. You can't get it out of your body. It's going to stay there for your entire life, and all that you can do is take steps to prevent yourself from developing shingles. Of course you can treat the rash and the pain. Other than what the doctor may tell you to do you can also apply a salve made of vitamin E and aloe vera. Separately each of these are used for skin problems, and are very effective. For shingles you mix a capsule of vitamin E and a tablespoon of aloe vera together and apply it directly to the area of rash and pain.

Vitamin B-12 has also been used effectively to treat shingles. Unfortunately it has only been tested with injections and it is not known if it is also effective if taken as a supplement or in food. Still it would not be a bad idea to increase your use of vitamin B-12 containing foods.

On the subject of vitamins, I would also increase my use of vitamin C and vitamin E foods. Studies of patients who were taking 1000 mg doses of vitamin C every 2 hours found a relief within 2 hours, and a disappearance of the rash within 3 days. They were also receiving 1000 mg injections of vitamin C at the same time, so I do not know if simply taking oral vitamin C will give you quite as good a results.

Vitamin E was found effective over the long run, when given for the pain that persists after the rash has disappeared. In the cases studied patients had been suffering for 13 and 19 years, and supplements of 1600 IU of vitamin E daily found relief after 6 months. If you decide to use this vitamin E therapy do not expect any immediate relief. Changes did not occur until the supplements had been taken for the full 6 month period.

SKIN PROBLEMS

Skin problems can range from acne, blemishes, wrinkles and spots to eczema, sores that won't heal, bumps and lumps, and all the way to skin cancer. The causes are many, but the underlying cause is often a lapse in your immune system. It isn't usually pointed out but your skin is your first defense against infection. The oils that your skin excrete are mildly acidic so that most bacteria that lands on you just dies. Other germs and poisons just lie there on the surface of your skin until you wash it away. Of those that get under the skin you can get rid of most of them by working up a sweat or taking a hot bath. In any case you can see that the health of your skin is very important to keeping your body healthy as well.

Once something gets through your skin it can get into your blood circulation and make you sick in a hurry. Viruses that normally cause you to have a sore throat, when they get under your skin they can be life threatening. It is always a good idea to look to the health of your skin to diagnose the health of your body. Aiming to keep your skin healthy, there are certain foods that are especially good for your skin and your body.

FOODS THAT CAN RID YOUR BODY OF SKIN PROBLEMS

The standard vitamins for general health of the skin are vitamin A, vitamin D, and vitamin E. Deficiencies of these vitamins produce diseases that show up on the skin, and taking supplements, or a diet high in them, heals many of the problems that develop with the skin.

Vitamin A is especially high in carrots and sweet potatoes, but is also found in most fresh vegetables. Vitamin C is the classic vitamin of citrus, but is found in much higher levels in rose hips. Vitamin E is found in wheat germ, whole wheat, and olive oil. While these foods will take care of the general health of the skin, for particular problems you need particular cures. Here are some fruits and vegetables for the particular problems of acne, blemishes, wrinkles, and spots.

FOUR FRUITS AND TWO VEGETABLES TO GET RID OF ACNE, BLEMISHES, WRINKLES AND SPOTS

A common vegetable, excellent in salads and used to make pickles, is also excellent against both acne and wrinkles. The vegetable, of course, is cucumber. The original remedy calls for liquifying the cucumber and using it to scrub your face each day. As an alternative just include cucumber in your diet.

Eat carrots for vitamin A. I have talked about vitamin A before, but not in relation to skin. Your skin has a great need for vitamin A, and a deficiency of vitamin A will show up as a disease of the skin.

Eat oranges for vitamin C. The health of your skin depends upon the function of vitamin C in strengthening the elasticity of your skin, and in assisting the transport of the waste products of energy from your skin to the outside of the body. Since each cell must use energy to live, each cell produces by products of its energy use. If these by products are not removed from your body you will be poisoning and polluting yourself.

Bananas are well worth using to banish skin problems. It is the banana skin that is used. Just take a banana, peel it, and apply the inside of the peelings to your problem skin areas. If you have a portion of your skin that is very difficult just secure the peeling over the area with some tape, and leave it in place for an hour.

Try strawberries for dry skin conditions. Strawberries are very easy to use. Just cut one in half and apply the raw areas to your skin. In the case of sunburn the pain should stop almost immediately, but with other more persistent problems it may take a while.

You can also use pineapple for problem areas on the skin. Take a fresh pineapple slice and use it to massage across the skin. It will help to clean the skin and neutralize fatty acids. You can even make a mask of the pineapple by taking a slice, pureeing it in a food blender, mixing the material with a little molasses, mixing it again in the blender, and apply the mixture to your face directly. This mixture should soak into the skin and help to cleanse it as well as to heal any current problems.

SLEEPLESSNESS

Sleeplessness is more often caused by worry and tension than by illness. Oftentimes when you lay down to sleep you can't rid yourself of the concerns and problems that you have had during the day. You just lie there awake, tossing and turning, and going over the same problems again and again. Of course you may also deprive yourself of sleep by drinking coffee, or some other caffeine drink, but at least then you know why you are having trouble getting to sleep. It is also possible to be so tired that you can't sleep quietly. Your body just will not relax and let you sleep.

Some of the popular ways of overcoming sleeplessness is reading and watching television. Both of these methods function in the same way. They make you forget your concerns of the day, and in forgetting your body relaxes and you sleep. I am not one of those people who falls asleep in the front of the television, although I know several who do. I often fall asleep in the process of reading. Sometimes I will go to bed just as tense as everyone else, open a book, and fall asleep before I have finished a single page. From long experience I can say that reading will usually put me to sleep within 10 to 15 minutes. On a rare occasion when I am either very tense, or highly interested in the story I am reading I may stay awake for an hour or more, but that doesn't happen more than once or twice a year.

People who fall asleep in front of the television always seem to do so while it is on, and they rest comfortably only so long as the television stays on familiar programs. Perhaps that is what wakes them up in the middle of the night, either an unfamiliar program comes on the air or the station they are watching has gone off the air altogether.

In any case food has always played a big part in putting people to sleep as well. Large meals make you sleepy, but they don't give you a good night's sleep. Going to bed slightly hungry is much better if you want to sleep well, and it is also safer for you. Still, in the light of feeling good, I want to present you with 3 foods that can help you sleep better. You may have your own remedies, but if they don't include the foods listed here, then give these a try as well.

THREE FOODS THAT HELP YOU SLEEP BETTER

The classic recommendation that a warm glass of milk will help you go to sleep, as it turns out, is true. Milk contains a small amount of the chemical tryptophan, which acts as a natural sleeping pill. Tryptophan is also found in turkey, but who wants to have a turkey sandwich before they go to bed. A warm glass of milk will not only give you a small dose of trytophan, it will also give your stomach something to digest, thus drawing some of the blood and oxygen from your brain. This combination is very effective in getting most people to sleep.

A popular folk remedy, that a great many people swear by, is lettuce. Perhaps eating a lettuce salad before going to bed will help you get to sleep, but the way it is usually used is to take a head of lettuce to bed with you. After you lie down just nibble on the lettuce for a few minutes and you should soon be asleep. If, by chance, you wake up in the middle of the night simply begin eating the lettuce again and you will soon be sleeping soundly. This is the story, and it is so simple that I think it is worth a try.

There is another very popular folk remedy that I also like. It is honey, and all that you have to do is take a tablespoon of honey an hour before going to bed. Those who use it say that it calms them down and relaxes them. Now honey is mainly just sugar, and taking the honey is going to raise the blood sugar level. But taking it an hour before going to bed will let the sugar in the blood both rise and fall, and perhaps it is that fall in blood sugar that helps you get to sleep. It sounds very reasonable and I see no reason not to try it. One caution, however, do not give honey to small children. Honey contain small amounts of bacteria that can actually poison little children, although there is not enough to bother adults.

SMOKING

Smoking will kill you. It killed my mother, and it has had a hand in the death of every life long smoker that I know of. It either promotes lung cancer, or contributes to heart attacks and strokes.

Smoking fills the lungs with particles and tars from the tobacco, and all of the toxic compounds in the smoke go into the blood stream. Since the lungs are the point in the body at which the blood becomes oxygenated, any gases which are very much like oxygen also go into the blood. Over a long enough period of time the body becomes poisoned, and the lungs become blocked with tars and smoke particles.

All of these compounds and particles in the lungs attack the little air sacks in the lungs resulting in a lot of bronchitis, and then destroying them causing emphysema. Then in other cases they simply cause cancer. The other poisons in the blood attack the blood vessels and brain and do their damage in those areas.

This is why doctor's will say that smoking shortens your life, and will result in a life time with much more illness in it. Now that more of the public is seeing the dangers of smoking more clearly there is a great interest in quitting, by more people. Since this is a book about the use of food to help you be healthier, I will discuss 3 foods that will help you control your smoking habit, and help lower your risk of lung cancer.

THREE FOODS TO HELP YOU QUIT EASIER, AND LOWER YOUR RISK OF LUNG CANCER

It is possible to quit smoking by eating carrots. After all, a carrot is a little like a cigarette, although it is what is in the carrot and not the way the carrot looks and feels that will help your quit. Carrots are good sources of vitamin A, and high levels of vitamin A seem to help relieve the craving for nicotine. The way it works is that you keep some carrots with you, and whenever you get the craving to smoke you eat a carrot instead. At the very least eat 3 or 4 carrots a day, and, so I have heard, you can usually stop smoking within about 2 weeks.

Another food that mimics the effects of smoking, helping you to break the habit, is sunflower seeds. Sunflower seeds release sugars into the blood and calms the nerves in the same way that smoking does. While you can use raw or roasted sunflower seeds, you should keep them with you and eat some each time that you get a craving to smoke. You should not only stop smoking, but you will get a definite nutritional boost from the sunflower seeds as well.

For the third food I am going to recommend broccoli. I have already mentioned it in relation to many other illnesses, and perhaps this will encourage you to actually put it into your diet. Broccoli is a good source of beta carotene, and studies in Japan have found that daily doses of beta carotene containing foods result in a great decline in all forms of cancer in current smokers. If you are still trying to decide whether to quit or not, or you are smoking and plan to continue, at least protect yourself with a daily dose of beta carotene foods. Besides broccoli all green and yellow vegetables contain beta carotene, and you should have one or more serving daily to protect yourself against cancer.

STAYING REGULAR WITH DIET

With the proper diet no one should have a problem staying regular. The basic needs are water and roughage. Of course you must also have a diet without any nutritional deficiencies, but most people in this country do that very well just by eating a variety of foods. The problem lies in our addiction to fats, sugars, and refined foods.

If your diet consists of refined flower in the form of breads and baked goods, daily amounts of red meat, fried foods, and regular visits to fast food outlets, I would not be at all surprised if you have problems of constipation and diarrhea on a regular basis.

However, if you diet includes fresh fruit or vegetables with nearly every meal, liquid on demand including water, and protein in the form of fish, chicken, and beans, I would be very surprised if you have either constipation or diarrhea more than once every 2 years.

Now, should you be having problems staying regular, but you don't want to change your entire lifestyle I can tell you my most sure fire remedies. To begin with roughage I prefer corn and onions. The corn I like on the cob, and one ear a day is sufficient. For onions, well I like onions, and I eat them raw or cooked. One medium onion a day works as well as an ear of corn. Other vegetables which get high ratings are sweet potatoes, broccoli, and asparagus. There is always something in season, and I like to eat foods in season as much as possible.

Potatoes are often recommended, although I see them more as a bulk food than as a roughage food. Oatmeal for breakfast is also preferred by many people, and although I don't have breakfast regularly I think oatmeal is a good choice so long as you don't load it up with too much butter before eating it.

For those of you bothered by problems of gas when you have meals high in roughage, don't let that discourage you. For one thing everyone has problems of gas no matter what they eat, they just don't think that it is bad unless it gets much worse than they are used to. It is true though that a high roughage diet will cause bothersome problems of flatulence. You can make a direct attack on the problem with a product called Beno, which is sold expressly to decrease the gas. There are probably a couple of other similar products around and you may just have to try them to see which works best for you. Otherwise I can give you hope. After being bothered with flatulence for several years, as a result of a high roughage diet, the whole problem had declined down to what it was when I was on the high fat, refined sugar diet. I don't know what happened though I have concluded that your body will eventually get used to the high roughage diet and you will no longer have gas problems even without Beno.

Fruits I love in season, and they do provide roughage, but I have never found them as effective as the vegetables I mentioned above. Even though fruit may provide roughage I think it is more valuable for providing enzymes that promote digestion, and high levels of vitamins that we tend to underuse in the winter. I am even half-way convinced that the reason many people feel better in the spring after a long winter is because they begin eating fresh fruits and correcting vitamin deficiencies.

Liquid intake is vital. If you do not get enough liquid your digestive system will not work properly. Water is probably the best source of liquid, although I also drink a lot of diet soda. For the most part I believe that diet drinks are a waste of money, and some natural foods people believe that they are also dangerous to our health, but so far I have had no problems and I monitor myself constantly. Fruit juices and milk are also popular, but they also carry a lot of calories. A healthy alternative could be herbal teas. With herbal teas you can also give yourself a vitamin boost, or medicinal treatment, at the same time you are filling your liquid needs.

Something I have not mentioned, but which should be, is exercise. Oftentimes the only change in lifestyle you will need to get regular is a 30 minute walk after each meal. You may also use a jog every other day, or a bike ride, or any exercise that makes you get out, breathe a little deeply, and sweat a little bit. The exercise doesn't have to hurt, but it has to make you breathe and sweat, and it should be done regularly.

STRENGTH

Strength is relative. If you are very young you are looking to getting a lot stronger, if you are in your prime you may want to improve, but mainly you want to avoid losing the strength that you have, and if you are older then you are looking for ways to recapture some of the strength you had in your prime.

Often strength escapes us quietly and silently. One day we are a high school or college athlete, and some other day we have been sitting behind a desk for 20 years and are beginning to have trouble climbing stairs. What happened?

Well, what happened was that we didn't use our athlete's

muscles for 20 years and they went away. We forgot that to get strong we had exercised and worked out for months at a time. And when we weren't working out to gain that strength and skill of body, we were still active working outside doing yardwork, or maybe in construction, or just walking and riding our bikes all over the neighborhood. We were never totally inactive for years at a time when we were young, and thats what it took to build the strength that we miss so much now. What can we do to bring it back to what it was 30 years ago? I will tell you some of my experiences since I have been hunting for the same magic formula, and at times I think I have found it.

HOW IT CAN RETURN TO WHAT IT WAS 30 YEARS AGO

Since we are talking about returning strength to what it was 30 years ago, let us assume that you are a man or woman over the age of 50. I will also assume that you have not exercised regularly for many years, and maybe not since high school or college. Therein lies the problem, without using your muscles they do not get stronger, or even maintain their strength. The saying of use it or lose it applies to muscles more than to almost anything else.

If you have truly been a couch potato for 10 years or more, and would like to regain your strength, I would advise a complete physical before starting. All the exercise books say the same thing, and with good reason. A physical will rule out most cases of heart disease or other underlying illness that could kill you or lay you up in the hospital before you ever begin. Ask your doctor straight out if there are any reasons you should not engage in an exercise program.

Now that you have passed your physical you have to make choices. If you like working out around people, and have some money and time, you can join a gym or an aerobics class. This is rather regimented, though they do have all of the equipment, as well as some instruction and assistance. Personally I would only be interested in going to a gym to work out if I was going with someone else.

For a more free and solitary beginning try walking. Recommendations for walking are that you start with a few minutes a day and work up to a brisk walk of 2 or 3 miles every other day. This is fine, if you have the time, and is probably the best method to start on, but it won't build much strength.

To build strength you have to use your muscles. Jogging, bike riding, working with weights, stairmaster, hiking in the hills, or building houses. To build your strength you have to use your muscles, and the more the better.

Once you are ready to begin a more strenuous activity, take your time. Never go out to climb a mountain, even if that is what you are aiming at. The same thing with weights. With weights begin working out with 20 pounds of weight, not 100. Give yourself time, at least a year before you start looking for results. If you have been inactive for 20 years, then give yourself 5 years to regain all of the strength you lost. You will be getting better every day, and you will probably never even know when you have surpassed your abilities of those earlier days. So long as you are in good health there is no reason why you can't regain lost strength, it you are willing to work at it.

STRESS

Stress comes with the package of living in modern day America. You have the stresses of job and home, and of school and relationships. Every year you face the stress of the IRS. Every single day there is stress of some sort, and on some days all that you have is stress. While most of us can live with the stress of our lives, there is always the danger of being overwhelmed by stress, and thereby reduced to hiding out to survive. In the hope that you never reach that point in your life, I offer some dietary methods of dealing with the stress of life and living.

Ginseng is the Chinese way of dealing with stress. A diet that includes 3 doses of ginseng daily enforces the immune system, and counteracts the effects of stress. Stress also depletes your bodies supply of vitamin A and vitamin C. Vitamin A is available in carrots, and vitamin C in citrus. Frankly, for a stress-ful life I would make good friends with all of the fresh fruit that I could find. Eat it fresh, in shakes, or cooked and mixed into pies or tarts. I have never yet seen anyone going through a bad state of depression who ate enough fruit. Come to think of it most people don't eat enough fruit at any time.

SWEETENERS

Sweeteners come in many shapes and sizes. The cheapest and most common is plain sugar. Sugar makes things sweet, but it also has rather a lot of calories, and contributes to tooth decay as well. As a result of interest mainly from those interested in diet several artificial sweeteners have been devel-oped. One of the first was sacchrine, which was followed by nutra-sweet, and several others.

It is not that these sweeteners do not have calories, it is just that they are many times sweeter than sugar so that serv-ings are much smaller. While you might get 10 calories in a sin-gle serving of sugar, you would only get one half calorie in a sin-gle serving of the artificial sweeteners. To correct one miscon-ception though, most artificial sweeteners come from plants. They are not just laboratory creations. Additionally, in the small quantities that they are used, most of these super sweeteners are perfectly safe. They are so sweet that it is unlikely that you could eat enough of any one of them to cause any side effects, though there is one exception.

WHY YOU SHOULD NEVER USE ONE OF THE MOST POPULAR

Several years ago now the sweetener sacchrine was linked to cancer in animal studies. It is in your best interest to use one of the other sweeteners than sacchrine. Since there are several choices available, and sacchrine is not the best tast-ing of the lot, it should not be difficult to choose something else as a diet aid. I will not say that it is the best, but nutra-sweet seems to have the flavor that is most like sugar.

TOOTHACHE

Toothache is usually related to tooth decay. The only permanent method of dealing with tooth decay is having the teeth drilled and filled, or else pulled. I prefer having my teeth repaired when I need it. This is based on general principles that I don't want to lose anything that I was born with, and on the general nutritional consideration that health tends to decline as teeth are lost.

Of course you may also have toothache in the process of dental work, or due to an accident to your mouth, or even as a result of some other illness or medication that you are taking. Toothache, for some, is not something that can be fixed but something that must be lived with from time to time. For these people, and even if it is just for the time it takes you to get to your dentist, you need to have a simple method of relieving toothache pain. Luckily there is a natural herb that is an excellent pain reliever for toothache.

A NATURAL HERB THAT CAN RELIEVE TOOTHACHE PAIN

The common household herb cayenne, as in cayenne pepper, is useful as a toothache pain reliever. When uncooked it is not hot, and it is very simple to use. Just rub the cayenne powder on the gums around the area of the tooth that hurts. It does take a while to work, and an application in the evening may not bring relief until morning. However, as a bonus to the slowness, cayenne can be used for any swellings and inflammations, not just those caused by toothache pain. Have a bottle of cayenne in your first aid kits as an emergency treatment for pains and illnesses of all sorts. If the pain is internal and not on the surface of the skin, take cayenne by the teaspoon, as much as once each 15 minutes, and you should soon have relief.

TOOTH DECAY

The only people I have heard of in modern times who did not experience tooth decay were native populations, before the white man brought them the blessings of civilization. Let's face it, our diet is lousy for preventing tooth decay. We have too much soft food, and too much sugar. I would think though that the major cause of our tooth decay is the lack of fresh fruit and vegetables in our diets. These not only provide nutrients, they also remove food particles from the teeth and gums. All of the attention we give to brushing the teeth is just an effort to imitate the natural teeth cleaning we used to get from our diet. Chances are we will always be subject to tooth decay, at least so long as we insist on eating soft foods and avoiding those that have some crunch.

PREVENTION WITH A SLICE OF THIS AFTER EVERY MEAL

Even with a soft diet you can help yourself with a slice of cheddar cheese at the end of each meal. The cheese not only helps to clean the teeth, but it contains enzymes that help to retard tooth decay. What is nice, when you are eating out, is that most restaurants have the option of fruit and cheese as an alternative to a sticky, sugary, dessert. It is also cheaper to have an apple and slice of cheese than a $6 slice of cake. If you decide that you want the cake anyway, then have a slice of cheese afterwards. It is also much more acceptable socially to eat a slice of cheese following a meal than to pull out a tooth brush and proceed to brush at the table. It is almost as much trouble going to the restroom to brush at the end of a meal, unless you are at home. Brushing your teeth is just not something we do in public, either in a restaurant, or at a friend's home. If it is not possible to have cheese at the table, take a couple of slices in your car and eat it on the road.

TOXINS

Toxins come at us in many ways. We have already looked at environmental pollutants as toxins, and what you can do about them. Now it is time to look at all of the other toxins you might come into contact with them and what you can do about it. Toxins come to us as contaminants of food every day, and foods can grow their own toxins if we aren't careful. We also introduce toxins into our own homes by the cleaning solutions we use, as well as poisons we may spread around to kill insects or unwanted weeds. You are also not free of toxins in the street. Many cities are plagued by smog, and the industrial toxins that abound in our cities may appear at any time. At least there are some foods that can purify our bodies and help to rid us of these toxins.

FOODS CAN PURIFY THE BODY AND RID YOU OF ILL-NESS CAUSING TOXINS

One of the prime vitamins to purify your body of toxins is vitamin E. Vitamin E, since it is a great antioxidant, prevents toxins from doing their damage while your body has the chance to eliminate them. Vitamin E can be found, in abundance, in wheat germ, sunflower seeds, and whole wheat. A n o t h e r vital vitamin to rid the body of toxins is vitamin C. Vitamin C is freely available in citrus, strawberries, and spinach. As you might have noticed by now, getting rid of toxins from the body is pretty much the same thing as strengthening the immune system. Besides vitamins C and E, a good immune system needs vitamin A (greens and carrots), and a good supply of zinc (which is available in turkey, brown rice, and spinach).

FLUSHING POLLUTANTS FROM YOUR SYSTEM

Flushing pollutants from your system requires two processes, control of what you eat, and an increase in what you drink. An additional act is the art of perspiration. Controlling what you eat means that you are going to have to fast from solid foods for at least 1 day, and preferably 3. This allows all undigested foods to pass through your body, and most of the toxins circulating through your blood stream to finish being digested, and to be eliminated.

You must, at the same time, increase your intake of liquids. However, liquids must be limited to water, herbal teas, or unsweetened fruit juices. Do not drink any beverages containing caffeine or alcohol, and do not drink milk or any beverage which is high in protein and sugars. With these drinks you can keep your vitamin levels high while getting rid of everything else in your body. These drinks will flush out your blood stream and digestive system.

You must also exercise sufficiently to produce a sweat, and preferably every day. It is best if you can exercise whenever you get hungary. If you can't then at least take hot showers frequently and exercise when you can. This will help to control your appetite and will cleanse your skin and the surface of your body.

You will probably feel like a new person in three days, but don't extend this plan for more than 3 days. Also don't do it more than once a month. You will probably lose about 5 pounds over the 3 days, but that will be mostly water, and you will gradually put it back on over the next 2 weeks. Overall it will do you good.

URINARY TRACT INFECTIONS

The usual symptoms of urinary tract infections are frequency of urination, and pain on urination. Either of these are a problem if you suffer from them. You can either urinate too often or not often enough, and pain on urination is a problem at any time. Urinating too often is not actually a sign of an infection, but may be a sign of diabetes, or some other disease affecting your body.

Urinating too little, in a man, may be a sign of an enlarged prostate or prostate cancer. It is can also be caused by bladder stones, for which the medical term is cystitis. Pain on urination can be caused by bladder stones, or an infection or inflammation of the urinary tract, called uritheritis.

If you have bladder stones the only remedy is to get rid of them. While that may require surgery, if they are small enough it may be accomplished with a highly liquid diet, and a device that breaks up the stones so they can be passed. These are medical procedures that your doctor will have to help you manage.

Bladder infections in general, cystitis, often respond to treatment with cranberry juice combined with a high intake of vitamin C. The prescription is to drink a glass of unsweetened cranberry juice every 2 hours while there is pain. You should also go on a program of 250 mg of vitamin C per day for as long as any symptoms persist. This is the best natural prescription for dealing with urinary tract infections.

ULCER HEALING

Ulcers often first show themselves as general pain on eating, burning pain in the stomach, and vomiting. You may think that you have stomach cancer, but it is more likely that you have an ulcer. And you may never know exactly why you have ulcers. People who respond poorly to tension, and who have a very stressful life seem to have ulcers more often. Smokers also have ulcers more frequently.

If you are like many people with ulcers you may resist going to a doctor for treatment and just go on a diet that includes a lot of milk in the hope that it will coat your stomach and reduce pain. Unfortunately the long term effects of ulcers, besides having the capacity of causing bleeding from the digestive tract and putting you into the hospital, also include weight loss and a general nutritional deficiency if you are unable to maintain a normal diet.

The best thing for you, when you are bothered by ulcers, is to control the symptoms as easily and quickly as possible, heal the ulcer, and maintain as normal a diet as you can in the meantime. The sooner that you get back to your regular diet the better off you will be.

In the light of those goals I would like to offer licorice, the children's candy, and what it can do for you, should you have the misfortune to develop an ulcer.

WHAT LICORICE CAN DO FOR YOU

Licorice is one of the most important herbs in Chinese medicine. It is used to cure all kinds of stomach problems, and is even added to other mixtures of herbs to make them easier on the stomach. Ulcers are just one of the uses for licorice. It is also useful for colds, the liver, to help remove toxins from the blood, and to treat glandular problems.

If you have an ulcer do not depend upon licorice candy for treatment. Licorice, as the Chinese use it, is in the form of powdered root. For this you need to go to a health food store or herbalist's shop. Either one should have a supply, and the cost is quite low. To use it for ulcers you should take small amounts in tea, but do not take large amounts frequently as it can raise the blood pressure.

VARICOSE VEINS

Leg pain is often accompanied by varicose veins because varicose veins are a sign of poor circulation to the legs. They are more frequently a problem of women than of men, although the causes are the same. Too much sitting and standing on hard surfaces, and too little exercise are the usual causes. The only solution offered by doctors are to cut them out if they cause too much pain and discomfort, and some people have it done just because they look ugly.

There are alternatives for treatment. Vitamin E, either in supplements or foods, is an effective treatment for the pain that accompanies varicose veins. Another natural remedy is to use a bayberry tea soaked towel wrapped around the portions of the legs with the varicose veins. Bayberry can be purchased at the health food store, or you may be able to gather it directly if it grows wild in your area. It grows as an evergreen shrub all over the east coast, and may have been carried everywhere else in the country as well.

To use a bayberry tea application dip a small towel or cloth in the tea and apply it hot to the legs. You can then cover this with a hot water bottle to keep it warm. It is even possible to keep this on all night if you can protect your bed from the damp towel.

WEAK IMMUNITY

I have already discussed various vitamins and minerals that are necessary to have a healthy immune system. The approach I would like to use this time is to give you some advice on foods that strengthen and promote the entire immune system all at once. They won't overcome nutritional deficiencies, but they will give your immunity a boost if your diet is close to being as it should.

The first food I would like to bring up is ginseng. Ginseng is particularly good for particular body systems, but its wide use in Asia is more closely related to its ability to boost the immune system. The cost of ginseng is not great, and it can be swallowed in a capsule or taken in a tea. In either form 1 to 3 doses per day are recommended.

Licorice, which I just mentioned as an ulcer medicine, also strengthens the immune system, and can be taken with most other medicines or foods. To use licorice get the root powder and not the candy. Use it daily in moderate amounts for best effect.

I would also like to suggest the use of garlic, or garlic oil, to strengthen the immune system. Garlic is used world wide for everything from infectious diseases to low blood pressure and lung diseases. Garlic can be taken fresh, as oil, or in tablets.

WEIGHT CONTROL

In other portions of this book we have covered all of the standard ways to lose weight: eat low fat high fiber foods, drink plenty of water, exercise, cut down on red meat, and eat fresh fruits and vegetables in season. However, even with all of these ways to lose weight, there are still behaviors that keep you from getting the control on your weight that you may want. What I will do in this section is to go over enough of the behavioral changes that you have to make to lose the weight you want, and to control the weight you have.

HOW TO CONTROL YOUR WEIGHT EVERY DAY

1. Do not go shopping for food when you are hungry. You have probably heard this before, but it is true. When you are hungry you are more likely to buy snack foods high in fat, which is not good for you anyway.

2. Find ways to make yourself exercise a little at a time. For years I have purposely parked at farther from malls and markets than I have needed to just to make myself walk an extra 5 or 10 minutes. These exercises don't hurt, but they do add up over time to thousands of calories burned.

4. Switch from regular ice cream to lite ice cream or frozen yogurt. The ice cream companies are getting so good with these that the taste is very close to regular ice cream, and you save hundreds of calories a serving.

5. Find something active to do rather than sitting around watching television every night. Dancing or bowling, or even miniature golfing, will cut down on your evening snacks and increase your metabolism. Do this at least once a week.

6. Set weight loss goals 5 pounds at a time. You may think that you need to lose 25 or 50 pounds, but no one has ever lost that much who hasn't lost 5 pounds first. Setting little goals like this also lets you go to a plateau and rest for a month or two if you want a break from dieting.

7. Avoid buffet meals whenever you can, and don't go to

buffet restaurants. This is difficult for Americans, who love the abundance of these meals. Unfortunately we also love to stuff ourselves with dishes we like at them. I promise you that you won't go home hungary if you stick to ordering your meals by the plate, you just won't be quite as full.

8. If you are a frequent user of butter or margarine find a lite brand that you like. While you can't use these for cooking or baking, they taste the same as the regular brands and save about 75 calories a pat. That can add up rapidly if you use margarine daily.

9. For desserts, make at least half of them fruits in their own juices. Fruit does not have fat, and when in its own juice it has no added sugars either. If you must add something creamy use fresh or frozen yogurt.

10. When you have your meals be reasonable in serving yourself, but take only one plate of food. I once lost 10 pounds over 5 months by doing this. It seemed hard to pass up food on the table, but the weight came off without otherwise thinking about it or dieting.

WORKOUT FOODS

An active person, who is working out frequently, has different nutritional needs from someone who is basically inactive. Activity not only burns calories, it also puts wear and tear on the muscles and bones of your body. Salts are excreted in sweat, and salts contain minerals. Vitamins are broken down and processed to rebuild tissue. While workouts are good for the body, if you do not have the proper nutrition and you are working out you can actually cause your body to break down. Some of the women who are in such excellent shape, and who run aerobics programs every day, actually workout so hard that they cause their bodies to break down. It isn't that they should workout as much, its just that they don't have the diet that they need to repair the wear and tear on their bodies on a day by day basis. Let's see if we can prevent that from happening to you.

FOODS THAT IMPROVE WORKOUTS AND SPEED RECOVERY

The first food that I would recommend is water. Exercise, and working out, uses up the body's water faster than it uses any other part of our nutrition. While we may have several quarts of water in our body, we can also perspire a quart or two of water every hour when working out on a warm day. For protection have a glass of water before your workout, have water available during and take sips whenever needed, and afterwards give yourself an hour or two to drink liquids to replace all of your lost liquids.

Complex carbohydrates are preferable to candy for sustained energy. It is much better to have a small plate of spaghetti an hour before a workout than a candy bar as you go out the door. By the way, the energy bars that are featured for athletes are based on complex carbohydrates.

Supplements are a good idea. A general supplement will make certain that your vitamin and mineral levels are maintained. Along with supplements you should also have your main protein meal the night before your activity, not in the immediate hours before workout.

As a last suggestion I would say that you should get adequate sleep. Sleep and relaxation allow the body to recover and rebuild damaged tissues. If you are cheating yourself out of needed sleep and pursuing a hard workout program you are going to break your body down rather than build it up. If you aren't certain how much sleep you need start with 8 hours and cut it down by 1/2 an hour each week until you feel deprived and sleepy during the day. Then lengthen your sleep by 1/2 hour. As you workout and get in better shape you will probably find that your need for sleep decreases, and you may even cut an hour off of your normal sleep pattern after a few months. But when starting out don't skimp or you could injure yourself and hurt your program.

WOUNDS

Wounds are the result of either accidents or surgery. Accidental wounds are dirty, ragged, and can remain untreated and open for hours or days. Surgical wounds are neat and clean, and will be sterile and closed within minutes or hours at the most. However, it is not the source of the wounds that accounts for their difficulty in healing, it is their nature in terms of how large they are and what damage they have done to the surrounding tissues.

Whatever the source of the wounds the first problem that must be confronted is bleeding, since most wounds bleed and bleeding will cause you the most immediate harm. In surgery doctors can pinch off, or tie off, parts of the wound that bleeds. This will get you through the immediate stages of the wound care, although other measures will be necessary very soon. In accidents you may have to rely upon simple pressure keeping you alive until the blood coagulates, or you get to a doctor who closes the wound properly. In either case you only have a few minutes if the wound is large and bleeding. At times of open wounds you do not want to rely upon aspirin as a pain killer. While aspirin works very well to relieve pain, it also acts as an anticoagulant, and will prevent your blood from clotting stopping to bleed. While this is good to prevent heart attacks, it can bleed you to death if you are bleeding badly.

Once the bleeding is controlled, the next problem is the healing of the wound. Some people have wounds that have refused to heal for years in spite of repeated visits to their doctors. You don't want to be one of these, and you can take a couple of dietary steps that might help to prevent it.

Vitamin C has been found to help wounds to heal. In fact vitamin C has been found to help wounds to heal that have remained open for years at a time. But for normal wounds, say for either surgery or accidents, increase your intake of vitamin C to at least 250 mg daily. You can easily get this amount from your diet if you eat high vitamin C foods. If you have a wound that refuses to heal increase your vitamin C to 1000 mg daily, and for that you are going to have to rely on supplements.

In some cases vitamin C is not enough. People with troublesome and unhealing wounds have been found to have low levels of zinc as well as a need for vitamin C. Zinc has been found effective in such cases as stubborn leg ulcers. If you have a wound, normal or otherwise, I would advise a diet high in vitamin C and zinc, as well as well balanced nutritionally.

One warning is in order. Before surgery doctors often advise a patient to diet. It has been found that the heavier the patient the more problems they have recovering from surgery, not to mention the greater difficulty they may have breathing and the extra strain on the heart. However, do not diet while you are in the process of healing. You can not be certain exactly which nutrients your body is in the greatest need of at this time, and you may slow your healing rather than help it.

WRINKLES

Wrinkles are the enemy of everyone who wishes to look young, and who doesn't? Wrinkles are not attractive, at least not when they dominate the face, but who are the victims?

The two largest contributors to wrinkles are the sun and smoking. Smokers will start to wrinkle in 5 to 10 years, usually around the mouth and eyes, and it will be progressive throughout the body after that. Of course with smokers you not only get wrinkling but also a darkening of the circles under the eyes, and an apparent loss of fat in the skin that leaves it looking dry. The sun does much the same thing, although the sun carries the added risk of skin cancer. However, a few years of good sun tans can give you permanent wrinkles by the time you are in your 20s. Is it worth it?

But the problem we are talking about is wrinkles. Besides the sun and smoking, nutritional deficiencies can also cause wrinkles. A vitamin C deficiency acts very much like smoking in causing wrinkles, and even fluoride causes wrinkles. This is too bad since fluoride also protects the teeth from decay. If you don't have a good diet for your teeth you may be faced with the choice of either keeping your teeth or getting wrinkles.

That is not much of a choice, and you would be better off having a good all around diet.

Other deficiencies that cause wrinkles are zinc, vitamin B-2, and fatty acids. These are all available in supplements or through diet. Nutrition must support the amount of moisture in the cells of the skin and the structure of the muscles and collagen in the skin holding it together to prevent and control wrinkling.

Think of it in terms of fruit. When fruit is fresh and growing it has a smooth and moist skin. When it has set around for a few days and lost some of its moisture the skin becomes wrinkled and loses it elasticity. This is the same thing that happens to your skin. If you allow your skin to become dry, which can happen when smoking constricts the blood vessels and prevents moisture from getting to the skin, it wrinkles. It can't do anything else since it doesn't have the underlying liquid needed to prop it up.

Having a deficiency in vitamin C, zinc, or vitamin B-2 works the same way that opening up a piece of fruit and cutting out part of the underlying structure does. When you do that the skin just collapses over the structure that is left. The skin may be perfectly healthy, but there is nothing to hold it out taught and it wrinkles. As a short term solution there are creams that you can use as you find the right nutritional diet to make your skin look the best that it can.

A FOOD BASED WRINKLE CREAM THAT WORKS

A wrinkle cream is something that will help you for a day or two, but which will have to be reapplied fairly often to have effect. It is not a permanent solution to a problem such as troubling wrinkles. For this reason I wanted to leave you with a wrinkle cream that is easily and cheaply available, and that you can do yourself without extensive preparation, or visits to pharmacies.

What I have come up with is a wrinkle cream based on eggs and olive oil. The procedure is to take the yolks of two eggs and beat them with 1/2 cup of olive oil. Brush this mixture over the areas of the wrinkles and leave in place for 10 minutes. Now beat the egg whites until they are stiff and apply them over the olive oil and egg yolk to make a facial mask. Leave the mask in place for 1/2 hour and then wash off with warm water and soft soap. By all reports this tightens the skin and rids it of wrinkles very effectively.

FREE BONUS REPORTS

FOODS THAT CAN CAUSE DISEASE

CONTENTS
What foods we over eat most frequently
Alcohol
Diabetes
Cancer
High blood pressure
allergies
salt

INTRODUCTION

Some foods have a much greater potential for causing disease than others. Most foods can cause disease only if taken in excess, although others are just as deadly as drugs or poisons to your body. Most of the time we get in trouble with our diets just because we eat too much and gain weight. In that sense many foods can cause disease, but some are certainly more dangerous than others.

WHAT FOODS WE OVER EAT MOST FREQUENTLY

It is easiest to overeat those foods that either taste good to us, or those that promote our hunger. Have you ever noticed that when choosing desserts you tend to pick ones that are really too big for you. I mean that if there are two pieces of pie available, one which is 1/5 or a pie and one that is 1/3 of a pie, you will choose the larger one whether or not you are hungry at the time.

This same force seems to take us over when it comes to taking servings at a buffet, whether it is in a friend's home or at a restaurant. While we may take small servings initially, we continue to eat until we can hold no more. The result of this is, not unexpectedly, that once we begin to gain weight we sometimes continue to do so throughout our lives.

Foods we overeat are usually desserts, such as pies, cakes, ice cream, and donuts. Sometimes we are driven to overeat meat or chocolate, and sometimes it is just alcohol that we can't control. I will save a discussion for alcohol until after we look at the others, since the dangers it causes to our health go beyond extra calories.

Pies, cakes, and so on all come under the category of sweets. The problem with sweet foods is that they increase our appetite so that we eat more of them than we should, have many calories, and have very little food value otherwise. The calories don't come from the sugar that makes them sweet, but from the oils that they usually contain, and that makes them satisfy our hunger.

Meat, especially red meat, is a very high fat food. Meat is also so easy to eat that we can have it every day in amounts that can easily add up to 1000 calories daily. Meat also has so much protein that digesting it affects our entire digestive system.

Chocolate comes under the category of sweets, but it also has the effect that it is addictive all by itself. There are many people who can get along on very little meat, and who don't care much for baked goods, but who eat chocolate daily. Chocolate is a very high fat, high calorie food with very little food value. It is said that chocolate turns on the pleasure centers of the brain, and in that way can act just like an addiction. Liking chocolate myself I can easily see how that might be true.

ALCOHOL

I thought that alcohol deserved it's own section since it is especially dangerous to the body. Alcohol in small amounts is not dangerous, however. Since alcohol can form out of any grain or sugar food there are probably traces of it in most of the fruit juices that we have, as well as small amounts in other foods.

Alcohol in large amounts is very destructive and danger-ous. You can't drive safely after more than 1 or 2 drinks, and chronically drinking large amounts of alcohol can result in dam-age to the liver as well as hallucinations and destruction of your social relationships. True alcoholics even develop cases of mal-nutrition due to neglect of their normal dietary needs.

DIABETES

Diabetes is one disease that is closely associated with diet. When diabetes occurs in young people, you don't worry about the cause, and most of the time you don't know why. But in older people you more often find diabetes in those who are overweight. In fact the heavier a person is the more risk they have of becoming diabetic. Often people will say that a diabet-ic person just ate too much sugar, although sugar is not a proven cause of diabetes. Fat is not a proven cause either, and we just have to conclude that it is something to do with the weight itself that contributes to a person developing diabetes. You should really be worried though if you are both overweight by 50 pounds or more, and there have been other people in your fam-ily who have had diabetes.

CANCER

Cancer is much more complicated in its relationship to food and diet. The strongest association with cancer is smok-ing. Smokers have more lung cancer, and more cancer of all kinds than other people, but there are also risks in our diet. Both fat and sugar have been studied as possible causes of cancer, and fat seems to be a stronger risk factor.

Other risk factors in our diet may be pesticide residues on vegetables. In South America there are high stomach can-cer rates in people who eat vegetables where the greatest amount of pesticides and fertilizers are used. This is not proof that these chemicals cause stomach cancer, but they might be a good argument for starting your own backyard garden.

The Japanese have lower cancer rates for most cancers than Americans. That is lower for most except for stomach cancer. Now since the Japanese are not known as a people who use a lot of fertilizers or pesticides it is thought that maybe their spices contribute to cancer. I would not say that this proves anything either. It is very hard to prove that a food causes cancer, and it could be just as well that the Japanese have something in their genes that causes stomach cancer as that it is their diet that causes it.

HIGH BLOOD PRESSURE

High blood pressure is associated with most of the death in the United States, making it our most common disease. It is not at all unexpected that it is also associated with poor diets, only the association is much closer.

If you do not exercise you will probably develop high blood pressure at some time in your life. If you do exercise, but you are overweight and you smoke you will still most likely develop high blood pressure.

As you get older, if you have had a good American diet, rich in meat and high in fat, your arteries are probably at least partly clogged with cholesterol. As they get clogged up the blood pressure goes up as well, and so does your chance of a heart attack or stroke from clots breaking off of the clogs and stopping the blood that flows to your heart or brain.

While you don't have to avoid red meat and baked goods entirely, it isn't a bad idea to find cholesterol free substitutes, and to keep your cholesterol intake under 30 mg a day.

ALLERGIES

While heart disease and cancer are the most serious diseases caused by food, allergies must be the most common. You can have allergies to most foods, although some are more common than others.

Allergies are peculiar though. You may have an allergy to milk and milk products, but if it is mild enough you may think that you just have an easily upset stomach. An allergy to milk usually shows up as diarrhea and vomiting. You could have one symptom or the other, or both. If your allergy is severe you will have an attack every time that you drink milk or eat anything with milk in it.

Allergies to eggs are also common, and it is also hard to avoid being exposed to egg containing foods. Even if you don't eat whole eggs, eggs are used in just about all baked foods, and even vaccines are grown in eggs.

It may be the acids, or something else in these foods, but allergies to tomatoes and strawberries can be encountered at any dinner party. Allergies to chocolate are also common, and they are even mysterious to those who do not share them. After all, there are so many people who are addicted to chocolate that it is inconceivable to them that anyone could be allergic to chocolate.

SALT

I have included salt as a food that causes disease because it is implicated as a dangerous factor in some of our most serious diseases. If you have high blood pressure you have probably been told to go on a salt free or low salt diet. When salt is digested its molecules enter the blood and make it harder for liquid to enter and leave the body. The result is that the blood pressure goes higher, and if you already have high blood pressure it can climb into the danger zone. On the other hand if you cut the salt out of your diet your blood pressure should go down.

If you do not have a blood pressure problem it still makes a difference as to how much salt you have in your diet. Even normal blood pressure will be raised if you have salt with each meal. Your body needs very little salt for its proper operation, and can easily get all that it needs from natural foods. It is never necessary to add salt to your food to get the dietary salt that your body needs.

It is probably a good idea for everyone to cut down on salt in the diet, and you might even find that food tastes a lot different than when it is covered over with a layer of salt.

HOW FOODS CAN HEAL

CONTENTS

Why we don't usually think of food as medicine

What we buy in the super market

Can foods really be used as medicines?

Where do we think that drugs come from?

INTRODUCTION

Foods can heal because most of our medicines originally came from the foods in our diet. Furthermore, many of our illnesses are either caused by dietary deficiencies, or else are made worse by the nutrients that we need to fight them. Because there are so many diseases and illnesses of different types it is necessary to know a great amount about both food and illness to be able to find the proper diet to either prevent or cure our medical problems. The Chinese have spent about 3,000 years trying to do this, and seem to have been about as successful as American medicine has been. That is not to say that all natural and food based treatments for disease are as good or better than the drugs modern medicine has developed.

It does mean though that there is a better diet to either prevent or treat every illness, and that increasing nutrients way beyond the minimum daily amount is sometimes necessary when we have certain medical problems.

Think of it in terms of what most women have gone through by the time they are 25 or 30 years old. Women in this age range become mothers, and when they are pregnant doctors prescribe special diets with extra vitamins and minerals. These are food based treatments for a medical condition that the entire medical community accepts. What I want to know is why they don't accept, with equal enthusiasm, that extra vitamins, minerals, or dietary enzymes, are just as capable of preventing diseases such as the flu, or colds, or cancer, or arthritis. I think that diet plays a part in all of these. If you don't have them perhaps you can prevent them with the proper diet, and even if you have, say arthritis, there must be a diet that is better for it just as there are diets that can make it worse.

WHY WE DON'T USUALLY THINK OF FOOD AS MEDICINE

Just look at the way medicines are packaged and sold. Not only are they put into little packages with labels in Latin, and all kinds of warnings about danger, but they are expensive, and you can't even get the best ones without seeing a doctor and getting a prescription.

Somehow this whole process just doesn't seem right to me, at least with the medicines that come from foods available in the super market. All of the vitamins and minerals that we need can be taken in the form of food. It doesn't matter if you are a vegetarian, or eat meat with every meal, if you eat a broad range of foods you are going to get enough of the basic vitamins and minerals to keep you healthy.

WHAT WE BUY IN THE SUPER MARKET

How do you go about choosing the food you eat every day? Do you plan out every meal using a nutrition guide, along with balancing calories and fiber, or do you eat mainly the foods you grew up with? Chances are that you eat what is familiar to you.

You know that some foods are good for you and some are bad for you in that they are high in fat, or they have a lot of sugar or salt. In general though, if you think about it at all, you believe that you have a pretty good diet since your American, or Hispanic, or Asian diet is basically good and healthy.

Actually you are almost right. Every cultures diet has both good foods in it, and bad ones. The red meats in the American diet have too much fat, and our baked goods have too much cholesterol. Asian diets are probably better, but it is disturbing that they have such high stomach cancer rates. Hispanic diets taste awfully good, but they are also high in fat and it is very easy to gain weight if you are eating large Mexican style meals as you get older.

On the other hand nutrition books list foods from each culture as being especially good to prevent different diseases. As you look at these nutrition diets you will see a different culture featured every month, or so it seems. One month it will be the beans of the Mexican diet, or the broccoli of the American diet, or the rice of the Asian diet. The truth is no one diet is perfect for everyone, and no single culture has all of the answers for all of our medical problems.

CAN FOODS REALLY BE USED AS MEDICINES?

The answer is yes, if you choose your foods carefully enough. There are two basic problems to choosing foods that will work as well as the medicines that your doctor recommends: the first is that you have to know what disease you are treating or trying to prevent, and the second is that you have to find a food, or foods, that you can eat daily to give yourself the nutritional boost that you need.

That is why so many people find that using supplements is easier for them than trying to plan a perfect diet that takes all of their needs into consideration. Many people resort to multiple vitamins that have larger than minimum amounts of all the basic vitamins and minerals. Lest you think that this is all you need, just remember that you can't live on vitamins alone no matter what the levels that you take.

Food has to supply not only vitamins and minerals, but fiber, and carbohydrates, as well as limited amounts of fat and salt. Bulk is what makes your digestive system work properly, and proper amounts of vitamins and minerals make everything else in your body stay healthy.

HOW DO YOU USE FOOD AS MEDICINE?

As I have said, to use food as medicine you have to know what you are trying to prevent or cure, and you have to know what is in the food that you are using. Therefore, there are 3 steps that you must go through: first, plan and use a good basic diet that will keep you healthy when you are well, taking into consideration any special needs that you may have. Second, learn everything you can about any medical problems that you have, otherwise you will not know what foods are required to treat what problems. And third, find out what the nutritional values are of the foods you eat, or that you are willing to eat. It doesn't do you any good to know that a particular food is the highest in a particular vitamin if you can't get the food, or if you wouldn't eat it if you could get it.

Planning a basic diet is perhaps the easiest part of using food to prevent illness. Every nutrition book will tell you pretty much the same thing: eat fresh fruits and vegetables with each meal, drink plenty of liquids, and make most of it water, eat meat sparingly, and keep your baked goods to a single serving, and not for every meal. Most of your calories should come in the form of complex carbohydrates such as potatoes, corn, rice, and pasta. Snacks should be limited to fresh fruits and vegetables. Limit caffeine and alcohol consumption to a couple of servings a day, and don't overdo anything. While this sounds very simple, it is, except that you have to do this every day and 1,000 times a year. Therein lies the problem. We like some foods, or types of foods, better than others. Some foods that we develop a taste for are the ones that we should limit the most. To that I can't really offer a solution, for the solution lies in self discipline and planning. You can plan all that you want, but if you lack self discipline you will repeatedly fall off the wagon. That is the story of most of us, over and over, and the only solution is to find out what medical problems result, how we should alter our diets to solve them.

Medical problems always have particular nutritional needs and therein lies the problem. We know that pregnancy requires extra calcium, and cancer can be fought with a healthy immune system. High blood pressure responds to garlic, zinc, and vitamin C. The problem is that we don't always know what is wrong with us, and dose levels of nutritional elements need to be adjusted just as often as dose levels of prescribed drugs to reach their maximum effectiveness. You will probably be unable to do this yourself, and most doctors won't take an interest in designing a diet to fight a disease if they are intent on doing it with prescription medications. It will probably be up to you, and to be successful you have to do some planning yourself. For one thing pay attention to everything that your doctor tells you about your medical problem. Always ask for full information about anything for which you are getting treatment. If your problem doesn't require medical management, then pay attention to your body. A mild case of arthritis will probably not send you to the doctor more than once a year, and even then he may not recommend a medication other than aspirin. For this case you can use nutritional therapies just as well, or better, than the medicines the doctor will prescribe for you. Of course if you don't know what nutrition is in food, you won't know what to use when you are ill, or even what to use to stay healthy.

No food is nutritionally perfect, and you can't eat one food every day even if your life depends upon it. This pretty well forces us to extend our diet beyond the one perfect food, should such a thing even exist. You have to know ten foods for each nutritional element, as well as which foods are high in more than one area of nutrition. Since you can't take pills to get carbohydrates and fiber you have to know foods that are high in carbohydrates and fiber are also high in vitamin C, or calcium, or vitamin A, or protein. With 20 or 30 ingredients to watch, and only a limited amount of food that can be eaten each day, how do you get all of each of the nutrients that you want every day, in 4 or 5 pounds of food. That is why the best diet, the medical diet, requires planning and study. At least you should know that it does exist.

WHERE DO WE THINK THAT DRUGS COME FROM?

It is only in these modern days that people have forgotten that drugs and medicines come from the foods we eat every day. Today so many drugs are created out of the laboratory which are mainly extracts from the common foods that we have sitting around in our kitchens, that we have lost sight of our bodies, and why the proper diet is important.

Today it is pretty common knowledge that penicillin comes from bread mold. At some time in the past the sick may have been fed bread mold when they were sick, and at least some of them were found to get better. Penicillin could easily have been discovered in that way although it waited for the development or biochemistry.

Natural food was also behind the discovery of vitamin C. Many years ago it was observed that sailors on long voyages got scurvy and lost their hair and teeth, except if they were given oranges and lemons. Eventually the active agent in preventing scurvy was found to be vitamin C, and after that people have tended to forget that it was the citrus fruits that helped us to discover vitamin C, and to prevent scurvy.

Food has been used as medicine over and over in the past, and it is only in the recent present that we seem to have forgotten that. All food is medicine, and some of it is good and some of it is bad. It is our job, if we wish to be healthy, to find those foods that keep us healthy and disease free, and to avoid those that make us sick, and that are responsible for the development of problems that lead to disease such as obesity.

HOW FOOD AND PSYCHOLOGY CAN WORK TOGETHER

CONTENTS

CAN Stress be controlled with diet?

What to do if you have a panic attack

Diet ideas for children you can't control

Personal stress test, how is your magnesium?

Do you have chronic fatigue, or housewife syndrome?   It might be your diet.

INTRODUCTION

Psychology refers to our feelings and thoughts, states of depression and happiness, and how we can go about solving our problems. Without the proper attitude it is impossible to get up in the morning, and with the wrong response to such conditions as depression we can end up eating ourselves into obesity. .

But food can be managed to solve these problems in the same way that they can be cause of them. If we know what we are doing, and follow the right suggestions, we can solve at least some of our problems with the proper meal, and that is what I want to talk to you about. I can't give you all of the dietary solutions to your psychological needs in just a few pages, but I can give you a few that might help and that is what I am going to do.

CAN STRESS BE CONTROLLED WITH DIET?

Stress is a problem of many sources. Of course it is psychological most of the time. Stress is usually about problems we anticipate, although it may also be caused by situations we are living through. But because stress is generally caused by outside forces there is no way that we can protect ourselves from ever coming under stress. It is more likely that we will have repeated stresses through our lives, with some more serious than others.

Whatever the source of these stress the way that our bodies react increases our physical need for some nutrients. Reinforcing these nutrients through food or supplements may help us to overcome the feeling of helplessness that often accompanies stress.

The nutrients found to be depleted in stressful situations include vitamin A, pantothenic acid (which is a B vitamin), vitamin C, and magnesium. While you may feel a lack of appetite in a highly stressful situation, you are better off if you can continue to eat a very mixed diet, whether or not the amount that you are eating is the same as when you are feeling better. Just as some people react to stress by overeating the wrong foods, others just stop eating altogether. Neither of these reactions is good, and each will lead to greater problems later on.

WHAT TO DO IF YOU HAVE A PANIC ATTACK

We don't usually associate panic attacks with food, but food and diet can influence them. Panic attacks don't have to have any particular reason to begin. You could be eating quietly in a restaurant one day and suddenly develop an overwhelming feeling of fear and depression. It may be a single event, or it might be something that is going to control much of your life for years to come. If this is the first time that it has happened you probably won't go to a doctor or psychologist, but if it has happened to you repeatedly you are probably looking for a way out. Before you try anything desperate, or commit yourself to a psychologists couch for 5 years, maybe there are some things you can do with your diet that can help.

Panic attacks, and such related problems as anxiety, depression, hyperactivity and learning disabilities all seem to have some relationship to your level of B vitamins. It has been known for a long time that B vitamins affect moods, and now it seems like the daily fluctuation of B vitamins in your diet can produce psychological problems. If you do not get your B vitamins to the proper levels in a very short time you might even consider that you have a severe depression complex and end up with years of therapy, and never really know the cause of it.

Treatment of panic attacks and depression with B vitamins takes very large doses. Luckily there is no danger of being poisoned by B vitamins, like there is of vitamin A, since they are not absorbed into the fat of your body. But that is for treatment purposes. For the everyday prevention of problems with mood swings, including depression and uncontrollable behavior, plan a diet high in the B vitamins. As an alternative take supplements. Either way the B vitamins may be your insurance against both depression and fear.

DIET IDEAS FOR CHILDREN YOU CAN'T CONTROL

If you have a child who is almost impossible to control, or you have to manage one, this section is for you. Children have been growing up in ways that their families hate for too long to remember. When these children have been tested, as occasionally they have been, for abnormalities in their blood many of them have been found to have just too much sugar in their bodies. As their body has tried to digest and process the sugar the centers for self control have been upset and these children have behavior problems.

Now if you know the eating habits of children, when given choices, it shouldn't surprise you too much that many of them end up with diets that have little more than sugar in them. Unfortunately sugar does not have very much food value. All that it delivers to the body is calories, just like alcohol. If you are a sugar junky and you are criticizing someone for drinking, you might as well criticize yourself along with the other person.

Now, back to children. The best move, if you can accomplish it, is to cut most of the sugar out of the child's diet. That can work if you have control of most of the meals and snacks that they eat. But if you don't you are unlikely to be successful in changing their eating habits overnight.

The alternative is to increase the child's intake of nutrients that will counteract the effects of the sugar. Studies of children's' behavior and nutrition have come up with two safe solutions that are well worth trying. The first is to use vitamin C in high doses. At least 500 mg per day rather than the 50 mg per day that are recommended to prevent vitamin deficiency disease.

The use of vitamin C is based on the idea that the uncontrollable behavior in these children is actually the result of an allergic reaction of the body to very high levels of sugar. Now whether this is true of most children who react to a sugar diet is unknown, but high doses of vitamin C were found to be effective in eliminating hyperactivity in about half of the children studied. This would give you about a 1 in 2 chance of correcting hyperactivity in children with nothing more than a few glasses of orange juice a day, and maybe a vitamin C supplement. Also, to be well kept in mind, vitamin C at these levels has no side effects and is not toxic.

It is also possible to attack behavior problems in children in a more direct manner. if you look at hyperactivity as a mildly out of balance chemical problem, then maybe it is possible to add a chemical or vitamin to your diet that will correct the balance. That is what vitamin B-6 may just be able to do.

Vitamin B-6 promotes the production of a chemical called serotonin in the brain. Serotonin acts as a natural tranquilizer, directly effecting the center of the brain that controls our moods and behavior. if you can control the serotonin levels in your brain you should never suffer severe bouts of depression, and your child should never have an episode of poor behavior in school or at home.

PERSONAL STRESS TEST, HOW IS YOUR MAGNESIUM?

If you suffer stress, and think that too many of the world's worries are on your shoulders, perhaps what you really have is a deficiency in magnesium in your diet. How can you tell?

Studies have found that areas of the world where there are high levels of stress related disease, such as heart attacks and strokes, also have very low rates of magnesium in the diet, and in those persons who are suffering stress. This is not proof, but if there is no danger to taking extra magnesium than it is certainly worth the trouble to find out if magnesium is a cure.

Our country is very low in magnesium intake generally. The best foods for magnesium that we have are legumes and nuts, and no group of Americans tested high in those 2 foods in terms of basics in their diets. We also seem to be a very stress oriented society. Have you ever noticed how stressed your boss gets if he can't find anything constructive to tell you. Maybe it is because of low magnesium levels that so many American companies rely on managers who want their workers to look busy whether or not they have anything to do rather than trying to find out what they can do that is constructive to the company? It makes sense in that way, though certainly not in terms of making the world work better.

In any case, if you are in a stressful situation you might look to the possibility of increasing your level of magnesium rather than taking aspirin or some other mood elevator. Magnesium, since it is too low generally in our diets, can be increased or supplemented without any danger to health.

To accomplish this you should increase your level to around 300 mg of magnesium a day, and you should use nuts or peas and beans to do it. If this is a problem, or you have any doubts then use supplements of around 200 mg. That should be sufficient to make up for a diet that is normally only around 100 mg of magnesium.

DO YOU HAVE CHRONIC FATIGUE, OR HOUSEWIFE SYNDROME, IT MIGHT BE YOUR DIET

Now everyone has suffered from fatigue from time to time. You just get so tired that you can't do anything, and that is just perfectly natural. But being that fatigued for an extended period of time, chronic fatigue, means that something is going on with your body other than just getting tired.

By the way, housewife syndrome is just another name for the same thing. Many wives, who are cooped up in their homes day after day, no matter how nice, eventually become so frustrated with the whole routine of cooking and cleaning that they develop patterns of fatigue. Sometimes this leads to having affairs, but it is much more likely to lead to a behavior that looks very much like chronic fatigue syndrome.

In any case it was found that supplements of B vitamins, iron, or folate were able to solve most of the cases of depression and chronic fatigue. Now I don't want you to think that nutrition is able to solve all cases of depression and fatigue. It can't because not all of them are tied up in causing these conditions in the first place. The problem with solving them is that they are not all tied up with something that psychologists can solve by having you lie on a couch and talking about your childhood either.

Depression, and any other behavior, is tied up with both the mind and the body. While one may be responsible for a condition in one case, and the other in another case, they are both affected. If you have a psychological condition for which a clear solution cannot be found, the source could be either the function of your body and mind, or it could be some event and activity in your life that is causing your symptoms.

Certainly it is good to make certain that all of your vital vitamin levels are up to normal should you become ill. This is true no matter what the source of your illness. After all, your brain chemistry, and vitamin and mineral balance will be affected no matter what the original cause of your medical problem. The only way to know is to correct any deficiencies that you have and see if the emotional problems persist. In over half of the cases psychological problems can be solved by diet.

I do not wish to run down the professions of psychiatry and psychology. After all, they are founded on a lot of research and study, and their theories are sound so far as they go. The problem with these sciences is that they do not recognize that there may be other sources to psychological disturbances than the mind. Why they cannot see that a person could be depressed by pain in their bodies I do not understand. Many times the pain that we feel from a disease is not aimed at the site of the disease itself, but at the body in general. When this hap- pens you have a situation where someone may have a mild ill- ness, but experience very extreme emotional or psychological changes to their behavior. The only, and best, solution to this type of problem is to find a combination of medication, psycho- logical treatment, and diet, that brings all of the imbalances into their proper ranges, and restores you to the levels of behavior that you need to be successful in your life.

Index

Order form for extra copies of FOODS THAT HEAL, for yourself or as a gift to a friend. Mail with payment to:

FOODS THAT HEAL
American Publishing Corporation
5196 Benito Street
Montclair CA 91763-5196

Please send _____ copies of FOODS THAT HEAL at $16.95 each postpaid

NAME
_____

ADDRESS
_____

CITY _____ STATE _____ ZIP _____
$ _____ Enclosed by _____ Check _____ Cash _____ Money Order

PS: We'd like to know what you think of this book to help us improve future editions. If we may use your comments in our advertising, please sign and date below:

Comments:
_____
_____
_____
_____

Signed: _____ Date: _____

Mail to:

FOODS THAT HEAL

American Publishing Corporation

5196 Benito Street

Montclair CA 91763-5196

OTHER HEALTH AND MONEY BOOKS

The following books are offered to our preferred customers at a special price.

BOOK   ### PRICE

1. Health Secrets $26.95   POSTPAID
2. Proven Health Tips Encyclopedia $14.97   POSTPAID
3. Foods That Heal $19.95   POSTPAID
4. Healing & Prevention Secrets $26.95   POSTPAID
5. Most Valuable Book Ever Published $12.95   POSTPAID
6. The Smart Money Guide $12.95 POSTPAID

Please send this entire page or write down the names of the books and mail it along with your payment

NAME OF BOOK_____PRICE_____
NAME OF BOOK_____PRICE_____
NAME OF BOOK_____PRICE_____
NAME OF BOOK_____PRICE_____

TOTAL ENCLOSED$_____

SHIP TO:
Name_____
Address_____
City_____ST_____Zip_____

MAIL TO: AMERICAN PUBLISHING CORPORATION
BOOK DISTRIBUTION CENTER
POST OFFICE BOX 15196
MONTCLAIR, CA 91763-5196